KERSHAW COUNTY LIBRARY
632 W. DeKalb St, Suite 109
Camden, South Carolina 29020
WITHDRAWN

Raising Healthy Cattle

by

WILLIAM T. TESTERMAN, D.V.M.
and
JAMES CARLSON, D.V.M.

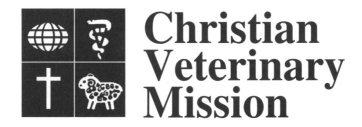

Christian Veterinary Mission

D1378700

Christian Veterinary Mission
19303 Fremont Avenue North
Seattle, WA 98133 USA
Current Book Information at:
www.cvmusa.org
PHONE: (206) 546-7569   FAX: (206) 546-7458

Copyright © 2004
Christian Veterinary Mission

This booklet, in part or its entirety, may be copied, reproduced or adapted to meet local needs without permission from the authors or publisher, provided credit is given to Christian Veterinary Mission and the authors.

These provisions apply provided the parts reproduced are distributed free or at cost—NOT FOR PROFIT. Christian Veterinary Mission would appreciate being sent materials in which text or illustrations have been adapted.

For reproduction on a commercial basis, permission must be obtained from Christian Veterinary Mission.

Library of Congress Cataloging-in-Publication Data

Testerman, William T.
  Raising healthy cattle / by William T. Testerman and James Carlson.
    p. cm.
  ISBN 1-886532-15-X (pbk.)
  1. Dairy cattle. 2. Dairy cattle—Diseases. 3. Dairy cattle—Health. I. Carlson, James, 1949- II. Title.
  SF208.T47 2004
  636.2'142—dc22

                                                                    2004026182

Raising Healthy Animal Series

Christian Veterinary Mission (CVM), in its efforts to be meaningfully involved in Third World development work, quickly found there was little appropriate educational material available. CVM set about developing basic resource materials in animal husbandry for farmers and agricultural development workers. Apparently, they met a real need, as these books have been accepted throughout the developing nations of the world.

The series of books published by Christian Veterinary Mission includes the following in order of publication:

Raising Healthy Pigs
Raising Healthy Rabbits
Raising Healthy Fish
Raising Healthy Cattle
Raising Healthy Poultry
Raising Health Goats

Raising Healthy Sheep
Drugs and Their Usage
Where There Is No Animal Doctor
Raising Healthy Horses
Zoonoses
Raising Healthy Honey Bees

As supplies are exhausted, they are revised before being republished in order to insure that they are kept current without compromising their simple, easy to read, well-illustrated style. All are in English, but it is our intention to publish these in other languages as soon as they are translated and the funds become available for printing. The Poultry, Rabbit, Goat and Pig books have been translated into Spanish and the Poultry book, in French.

In addition to the above, the following books are in varying stages of development:

Slaughter and Preservation of Meat
Buffalo Husbandry

CVM fieldworkers have also developed specific training materials for the countries in which they work.

Christian men and women, in a labor of love and service, for people in need throughout the world, have put all of these books together. It demonstrates dedication to their profession, service to humanity and a witness to their faith. We hope that they are a help to you in developing an appropriate livestock program to meet your needs. We pray God's blessings on their use.

They may be ordered by e-mail:
wharsh@cvmusa.org or by phone, 206-546-7368.

Leroy Dorminy
Founder, CVM   E-mail missionvet@aol.com

THE AUTHORS

James Carlson, D.V.M. graduated from Colorado State University College of Veterinary Medicine in 1974. He and his wife Pat have three children, Kristen, David, and Jeffrey. Dr. Carlson had a mixed practice in Julesburg, Colorado from 1974 to 1990. Since then he has been involved in a family ranching and farming business, as well as doing part time feedlot consultation. He and his wife have made numerous trips to Haiti and also Kenya on short term missions.

WILLIAM T. TESTERMAN, D.V.M., graduated from the school of veterinary medicine at Auburn University, Auburn, Alabama, in 1970. Following two years as a veterinarian with the U.S. Army, He served two years in the Peace Corps in Peru working with an artificial insemination project. After eight years of mixed practice in Tennessee and Washington, he returned to Bolivia for another two years with Christian Veterinary Mission with his family, where he helped develop a hands-on teaching experience for veterinary students in the Bolivian University. He has continued working in a mixed practice in Anacortes, Washington where he lives with his wife Ann. They have three daughters Shelly, Jill, and Nora.

ACKNOWLEDGEMENTS

A special thank you goes to the following individuals for their contributions to the cattle book.

For review of the written material and technical suggestions, thanks goes to the following persons: Leroy Dorminy, D.V.M.; Kenneth Weinland, D.V.M.; Jerry Olson, D.V.M.; Warren Wilson, D.V.M.; David E. Bartlett, D.V.M.; Larry Campbell, D.V.M.; and Jim Collier. Shelly Randall reviewed and made corrections in the initial manuscript and Kelly Ward, D.V.M. performed the final editing and made valuable suggestions to improve the content of the material.

A picture is worth a thousand words and the book has been improved a thousand-fold from the talent of the artists who contributed their time and effort. A special thank you to Linda Schneider, Nancy Haugan, D.V.M., Todd Cooney, D.V.M., and Marian Bowser.

For our family and friends, we appreciate your patience and support while working on the manuscript. Without your encouragement, the project would have never been completed.

TABLE OF CONTENTS

Section I

Cattle Production

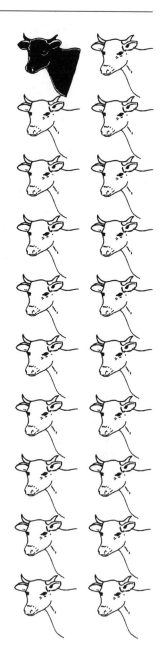

INTRODUCTION

As one of our earlier domesticated animals, cattle have given us many reasons to value them. They have been a human companion for 8,000 to 10,000 years. While we sleep at night, they are at work gathering foods, non-digestible for us, and turning it into useful nutritious products.

A more marvelous food factory cannot be found especially one with such wonderful by-products. When adequately fed and cared for, cattle are very productive under a wide range of conditions and environments. Meat, milk, butter, cream and cheese are the most obvious gifts from our four-footed friends, but there are many more. We harvest bounty from them in the form of food for the table, leather for our clothes and shoes, fertilizer for the soil, glue for industry, and even combs for our hair.

Cattle help to conserve soil through their grazing nature and production of manure. Over the years, the economic well being of humans tends to rise wherever cattle are found. Historically, man has migrated more in search for food for his cows than for any other reason, resulting in the settling of new frontiers

A brief introduction to the importance of cattle production and its role in providing nutrition follows for the interest of the reader. The most important by-products of milk are also discussed with a special emphasis placed on the manufacture of cheese

Treatment and care of cattle is only possible when they can be carefully observed. In order to closely work with them, they must be restrained. Once under control, proper examination for illness or related problems can be made, as well as administration of medications. Restraint and handling is discussed early in the book to allow the reader to become familiar with these techniques.

Following restraint, a section of the book will cover management, nutrition and feeding practices, along with a discussion on health and disease problems. Reproduction, an important part of dairy cattle production, will be included as well as an introduction to the art and practice of artificial insemination. Mastitis will be given special attention due to its economic importance in the dairy cow.

There are many aspects of cattle production that are not covered in this book due to restrictions on space. The reader is referred to related literature for further research in areas of interest. It is hoped that the material presented will provide a beginning point for those interested in raising cattle for the many benefits they may provide.

IMPORTANCE OF CATTLE

Ruminant animals, which include beef and dairy cattle, have an important role in feeding the world because of their unique ability to convert roughage and concentrates into nutrients that are edible for humans. Even though a large part of the world is not suitable for the production of grains, these lands may grow forage crops that cattle can utilize.

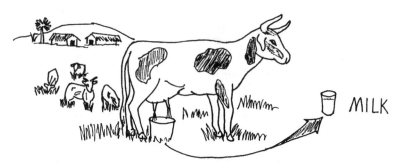

Cows graze to produce dairy products.

Milk and meat are the two most important food items that come from cattle. Milk can be processed into related nutritious products such as butter, yogurt, and cheese.

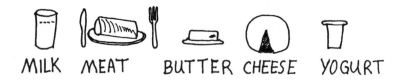

MILK   MEAT   BUTTER   CHEESE   YOGURT

One can only realize the benefits of milk if the dairy cow produces more milk than is necessary to raise her offspring. An exception can be made if artificial milk is used to raise the newborn calf.

Dairy production has a large labor requirement compared to other livestock enterprises. In addition to milking the cows twice a day, there are demands for handling, feeding, removal and disposing of manure, and care of the replacement stock. In many areas of the world there is an abundance of labor that can be used by a group or village dairy operation.

The amount of land required for a dairy unit which includes the cow and replacement heifer, varies widely. In areas with little rainfall, up to

10 acres may be needed per unit. In other areas that can produce cultivated crops to provide forage and grain for the cow, the requirements could be as low as 2 to 3 acres per dairy unit.

Milk is an almost perfect food for human consumption since it has a high level of available nutrients. However, bacteria can grow well in milk when it is not kept at a cool temperature. Even when milking is performed in a very clean manner, bacteria will still be present since they occur normally inside the udder of the cow.

Bacteria from the environment may be introduced as contaminants during milking, storage, and transport. When the temperature of the milk rises above 50 degrees Fahrenheit (10 degrees Celsius), bacteria begin to multiply very rapidly. Although some of the bacteria will cause no harm to humans, others can produce disease. All bacteria will have an effect on the physical qualities of milk if allowed to multiply, by causing it to sour or producing unwanted flavors.

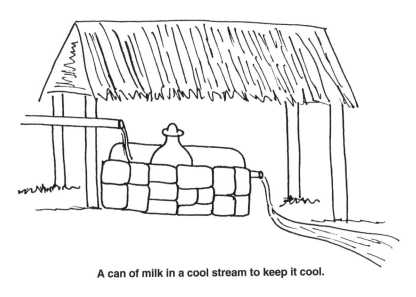

A can of milk in a cool stream to keep it cool.

One way to kill the harmful bacteria in milk is to heat it to a certain temperature and hold it there for a specific period of time, a process called pasteurization. This is usually accomplished by heating it to 161 degrees Fahrenheit (71.6 degrees Celsius) for 15 seconds. This is often referred to as "flash" pasteurization or short time high temperature pasteurization. Another method, referred to as "batch" pasteurization, is also effective. In this process the milk is heated to 145 degrees Fahrenheit (62.7 degrees Celsius) for 30 minutes. Batch pasteurization is often used in small dairies and for home use.

Milk being heated to kill the harmful bacteria.

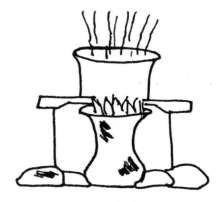

Both "flash" and "batch" pasteurization will destroy all known human milk-born disease organisms, and will decrease other bacteria levels normally found in milk, resulting in an increased shelf life. Important nutrients are not destroyed in the pasteurization process. Although enzymes will be inactivated by the heat treatment, they are not necessary for human digestion. The important sources of protein and calcium in milk are not altered by the pasteurization process.

In summary, pasteurization of milk is a very important process in which disease-causing bacteria are destroyed. The procedure is not costly to perform, the milk's nutritional value is not altered, its shelf life is increased, and the safety of the milk for human consumption is assured.

Cheese, yogurt, buttermilk, cottage cheese, and butter are important products which can be manufactured from milk. Where transportation of fresh milk is difficult or facilities are not available to keep the milk cool, processing the milk into alternative products is an effective way to preserve the nutrients. It is also a way to expand the market potential of milk.

The food products cheese and yogurt are the result of selected strains of bacteria converting the milk protein, casein, into an altered form. Commercial cultured buttermilk is prepared from skim milk that has had a starter culture of bacteria added, and has been allowed to ferment until the desired changes occur. Yogurt is produced in a similar way, but by using the activity of different cultures of bacteria. Cheese, likewise, is the result of selected strains of bacteria introduced to milk which produces a curd, a process in which solid particles of milk settle out. After the removal of moisture (whey) and addition of salt, the curd is allowed to ripen by the action of other bacteria which gives a particular flavor and form to the cheese. It is important to keep the temperature and humidity at constant levels during the ripening process.

Meat comes from cull cows and the excess male offspring. It can be prepared in a variety of ways for human consumption. In areas without refrigeration, the storage of fresh meat can be a problem. Drying is the most widely used method to conserve meat.

In summary, the production of meat and milk from cattle is very important in providing food for local consumption, and economic improvement for a farmer and his community. The means to increase the potential of the cattle herd will be explored in the remainder of this book. It is hoped that a foundation will be presented which will lead to increased knowledge for the management of a successful cattle farm.

Section II

Facilities and Handling

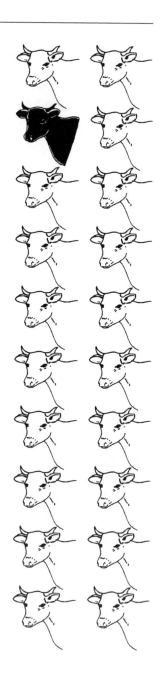

CONTROL AND RESTRAINT OF ANIMALS

CONTROL

When working with animals, it is important to have provisions to handle them and to provide adequate protection from the environment. Some animals are grazed on open range conditions. This type of operation can be used for young stock and heifers, but has drawbacks for a dairy herd. When the animals are not seen nor handled every day, they develop a fear of man. It is also hard to check for signs of disease and other problems.

Controlled grazing is better suited for cattle operations. The two most common methods are by herding or fencing. In herding, the cattle are moved from place to place for grazing and water. The herder most commonly controls the cattle either on foot or by using horses. By using fenced pastures, the animals are held within a certain area. The fences may be made of locally available materials such as thorn bushes, split logs, whole saplings, strand wire, woven wire, or lumber.

While fencing decreases the manpower needed to control cattle, it is expensive to build even when local materials can be used. Using thorn bushes can serve as a temporary method to control cattle. It is not strong, but can used on a temporary basis.

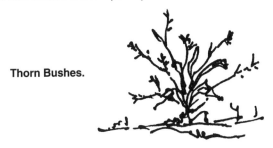

Thorn Bushes.

Whole saplings can be used for fencing by lashing or nailing them together. The saplings for the cross support section should be about 2-3 inches (5-8 cm) in diameter and 6-8 feet (2-3 meters) long. The crosses can be from 8 to 16 feet (2 1/2 to 5 meters) apart depending on the strength desired. The horizontal pieces should overlap by 2 or 3 times the width of the support X. This fence is more permanent and can take moderate pressure by cattle.

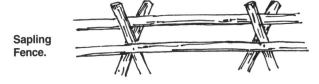

Sapling Fence.

A split rail or pole fence is made of heavier materials than the sapling fence. It consist of putting rails (split logs) of top of each other in a zigzag fashion. The poles of logs should overlap by 1-2 feet (1/3 to 1/4 meter) at each crossing.

Split Rails.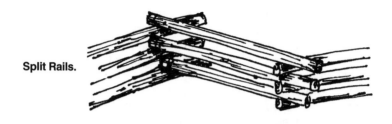

A vertical post driven into the ground at each crossing point will give added strength. Round poles will have to be lashed or nailed together. If split logs are used, lashing or nailing will give added strength but can be omitted, This is a sturdy fence and lasts a long time if rot resistant wood is used. It withstands cattle pressure very well except that it generally cannot be built tall enough to be cattle proof.

A board fence is probably the strongest fence designed for cattle. It consists of upright posts set in the ground with boards nailed to them. The strength of this fence can be increased by using heavier boards and setting the posts deep in the ground. It is very strong and can be built as high as necessary to be cattle proof. A disadvantage is that it is expensive to build and thus to control costs, it is usually used only for corrals or handling areas.

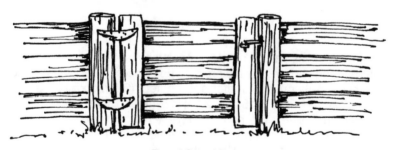

Board Corral Fence.

When available at a reasonable price, wire fencing is an excellent method to control cattle. Metal or wood posts are set in the ground and the wire is attached to the post. Depending on the number of wires used (usually 3 to 6), the fence can be very, cattle proof.

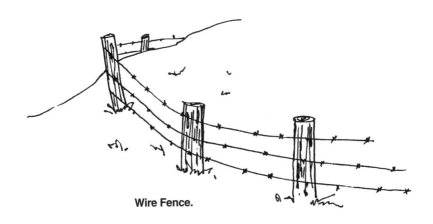

Wire Fence.

A method to control animals in close quarters should include shelter and facilities for protection. In most cases a simple structure to protect animals from the sun may be all that is needed. If weather conditions are severe, more care should be taken for adequate protection. Young animals should have special attention as they are more susceptible to weather changes. Protection during milking time along with a method for holding the head of the cow while milking is very helpful.

RESTRAINT

Restraint is a very important consideration when working with animals. When procedures such as giving injections, dehorning, vaccinating, caving assistance, or blood testing are performed, some method must be used to keep the animals still. The methods used must be safe both for the animal and the handler.

In general, cattle should be restrained as little as possible to get the job done. Since they are usually worked with on a daily basis, they should require less restraint, but like any animal they are afraid of the unknown and can become very excitable. When using any type of restraint, the operator should use caution as well as good judgment.

In restraining animals, techniques that divert their attention are very useful. This is accomplished by causing temporary pain in one part of the body which takes the animal's attention away from the area being treated.

The tail restraint is a common way of diverting the cows attention. The operator should place his hands close to the base of the tail to avoid breaking any bones and should stand to one side to avoid getting kicked by the cow.

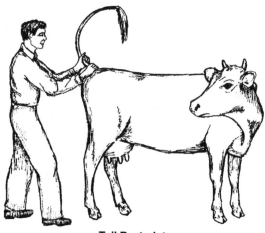

Tail Restraint.

A nose lead is another simple way to control animals. Many procedures can be performed such as injections, hoof examination, or minor surgeries by applying pressure to the nose using a suitable nose lead.

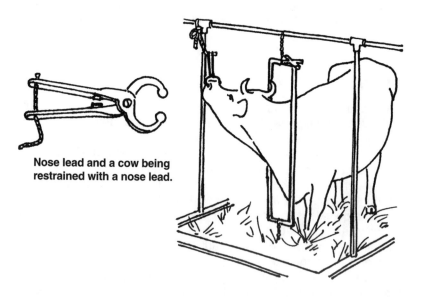

Nose lead and a cow being restrained with a nose lead.

When a nose lead is not available, manual pinching of the nose will often be enough to restrain the cow for brief periods. The nose is grasped with the thumb and forefinger of one hand while the other hand is used to hold the ear or horn for stability. This can be difficult if the animal is very strong, but may be useful in an emergency.

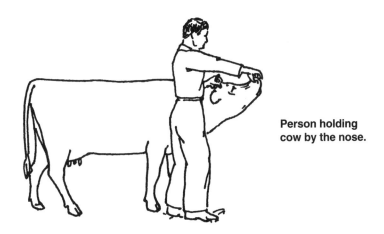

Person holding cow by the nose.

A rope halter is often used as the only means to hold animals. A rope and metal ring can make a very effective halter. The rope is spliced to the metal ring and a bight of rope is passed through the ring forming two loops, a larger one which is passed around the head and a smaller one which goes around the nose. When the rope is pulled, pressure is applied on the nose and provides the restraint needed.

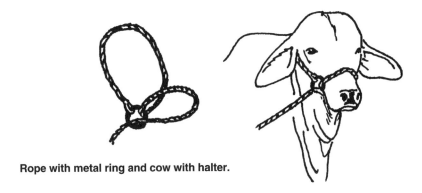

Rope with metal ring and cow with halter.

If a metal ring is not available, a rope fastened around the animals neck with a knot that will hold fast can be used. A bowline is a very useful knot for this purpose. It will not slip when pressure is applied which avoids choking the animal. To make a bowline, take the standing part of the rope in the left hand. The end, held in the right hand is then laid on top of the standing part and grasped with the thumb and the index finger, the thumb being underneath. Next, it is twisted up and away from the body and the end is passed through the loop, around the standing part and down again through the loop.

21

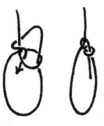

A bowline being tied.

Once the knot is tied around the animals neck, a bight in the standing part is passed through the loop and over the nose to complete the halter.

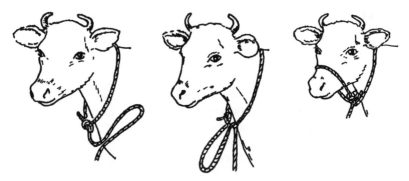

Rope halter, loop, and completed halter.

Casting an animal to work on their feet or perform other functions is often necessary. The standard method of doing this is called the rope squeeze. After securing the animal with a strong halter, a rope is passed around the head and a loop is made using a bowline knot as indicated in the drawing.

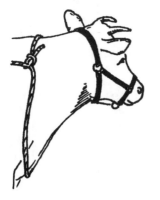

Loop over the neck.

The rope is then thrown over the back to the opposite side as indicated.

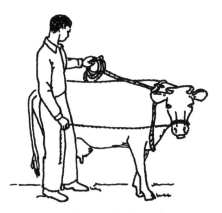

Reaching under the cow, the rope is brought up around the body and under the standing part of the rope near the bowline to form a half hitch just behind the shoulder.

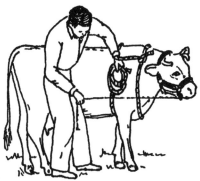

By putting the end of the rope over the cow's back again, another half hitch is made just in front of the udder or prepuce completing the tie. By pulling on the rope the cow will be forced to lie down.

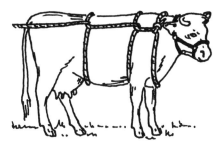

The rope squeeze can also be used in a variation of the above technique. After securing the animal with a halter, instead of placing the loop around the neck, a tie is made around the horns using a bowline.

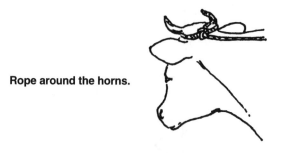

Rope around the horns.

The half hitches are then performed the same as in the other rope squeeze, behind the shoulder and in front of the udder or prepuce.

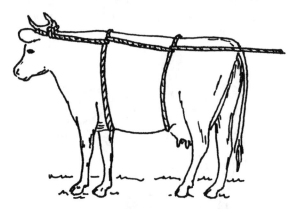

Rope squeeze with rope around the horn.

An alternative method of casting devised by Dr. D. R. Burley, called the Burley Method has several Advantages. For one, it is not necessary to tie the rope around the horns or the neck. It is simply passed around the animal's body which takes less time. Second, this restraint does not put pressure over the thorax avoiding damage to the lungs and heart. Third, the udder on cows and the prepuce of bulls are avoided. Also, after the animal has been cast, both rear legs can be tied with the ends of the casting rope.

After the animal has been secured with a halter, a long piece of rope (12 meters) is placed over the back with its center at the withers. Both ends are placed between the forelegs and crossed at the chest. One end is carried up each side of the animal's body and the two are crossed again over the back. Each end passes downward between the rear legs passing between the inner surface of the legs and the udder of scrotum.

24

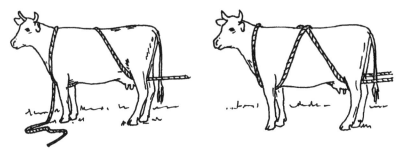

Beginning and ending of applying the Burley casting method.

When the ends of the rope are pulled the cow will lie down. The direction may be controlled somewhat by pulling the casting ropes to one side or the other.

One of the advantages of this method is that the rear legs may be tied using the ends of the casting rope. To do this, the rope is kept taut, the rear leg is pulled upwards, and a half hitch is placed around the fetlock.

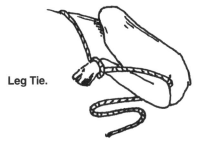

Leg Tie.

To secure the leg, the end of the rope is carried around the leg and hock, then back under the leg, and wrapped around the fetlock. Several such wraps may be made for added security.

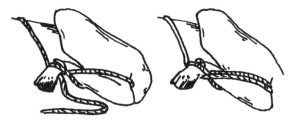

Figure 8 tie.

By using these restraint methods the risk of injury can be decreased to both the animal and operator. It is important to practice these techniques before you need to use them to avoid unexpected problems.

Section III

Digestion and Nutrition

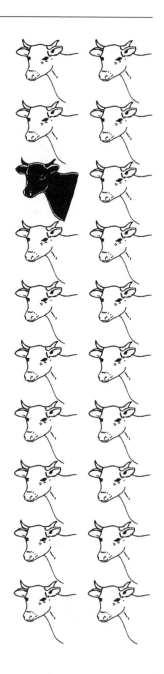

NUTRITION AND RATION FORMULATION

Nutrition is one of the most important aspects of beef or dairy production. An undernourished cow will not produce milk or beef, nor will she reproduce. Without these two functions, a dairy program will not be successful. To understand nutrition, a review of the digestive system of the cow is important. Cattle, like other ruminants, are multi-stomached animals. They are cloven-hoofed, and chew their food again after it is swallowed. Because of their unique digestive system, they can convert low quality, high fiber food into digestible nutrients for humans. This is made possible by the large fermentation vat called the rumen, the first of the four stomachs in the ruminant animal.

When the food is initially chewed and swallowed, it is greatly reduced in particle size, and mixed with enzymes in the saliva. Once in the rumen, additional fluids are added to the fibrous material to soften and enhance the digestion process. More resistant plant material are returned to the mouth to be chewed again, a process known as "cud-chewing."

Once the food is mixed and prepared in the rumen, fermentation takes place to produce usable materials for the body. The process of fermentation is a complex metabolic function which is aided by millions of bacteria and protozoa, rumen fluids, a desirable temperature, and a constant mixing of the material by muscular contractions of the rumen.

The micro-organisms which break down the food particles use some of the energy for their own growth, while other nutrients are converted into soluble forms, which are absorbed into the blood stream. Any undigested food continues on to the reticulum (honeycomb), omasum (book), abomasum (true stomach), and small intestine, where the process of digestion is completed.

Proteins, fats, and carbohydrates are changed into simpler substances which can be absorbed into the blood stream and used for growth and milk production. Any material not broken down in the digestion process is passed through the cecum, colon and rectum where it is excreted.

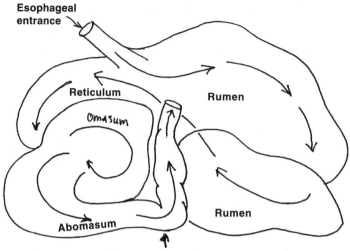

Esophageal entrance

Reticulum

Omasum

Rumen

Abomasum

Rumen

Leaves to small intestines

Stomachs of the rumen showing direction of the flow of food.

NUTRITION

The basic elements of nutrition are found in:

1) Water
2) Energy (Carbohydrates and Fat)
3) Protein
4) Vitamins and minerals

Water makes up over one-half of the total body weight. It is essential for the many complex processes that occur in the body. An animal's feed intake is related to the amount of water consumed. If water consumption decreases, the feed intake will be less than normal. An average animal should drink:

1-1.5 gallons of water/100 lb. body weight per day or

4-6 liters of water/50 kg. body weight per day.

Depending on the air temperature, humidity, feed source, age, body size, activity level, and the quality of the water, the water consumption will vary. Young moist plants may contain up to 90% water while older mature plants may have only 10% moisture content. Animals fed a dry forage need more fresh water to meet the daily requirements than those grazing green pastures. Animals receiving less water than required will eat less feed, their blood will thicken, and their performance will decrease. They may eventually die from dehydration. Zebu cattle, because of their adaptation, require less water than European cattle. At least two times a day, cattle should be allowed free access to water.

Estimated Daily Water Needs of Cattle

Species	Weight (kg)	Condition	Approximate daily water needs (liters)
Cattle	50	Growing	5 to 6
	100	Growing	8 to 9
	150	Growing	12 to 14
	200	Growing	17 to 19
	300	Growing	23 to 25
	450	Fattening	30 to 34
	450	Pregnant	30 to 38
	550	Lactating	38 to 50
	500	Grazing	20 to 30

The body receives its fuel from the energy found in food. It can be compared to the gasoline that makes an engine run. Without energy, the animal cannot walk, grow, reproduce, produce milk or meat or even breathe. This energy comes from the breakdown of carbohydrates and fats found in the consumed feed.

Carbohydrates are composed of fiber, starches, or sugars. The body is able to produce heat and energy from the breakdown of these substances. If excess carbohydrates are taken in, they will be stored in the body as fat.

Fat is most often found in the form of plant fats such as soybean oil, peanut oil, or in animal fats such as tallow and fish oil. More energy is found in fats than carbohydrates on a per gram basis. In addition to providing energy, fat serves as a protective covering for the internal organs and as insulation for the body.

In order to make muscle tissue, milk, and to repair the body, protein is necessary in the diet. A young animal has a greater need for protein than an adult because it is building muscle and other tissues at a greater rate. Likewise, a pregnant cow needs extra protein for the developing calf, and to supply extra milk for her offspring.

Protein comes from two main sources, grass or hay, and supplements which can be added to the feed. Young animals receive their protein from milk. When excess protein is taken into the body, it will be used as energy. Urea is a product that animals can convert into a usable high quality protein, however it requires energy such as that found in grains for the conversion. Without a high energy source such as grains, urea can be toxic to livestock.

For healthy bones and teeth, minerals are necessary in the diet. They are also essential for healthy muscles and for maintaining the balance of fluids in the body. Plant materials supply most of the minerals but occasionally supplements need to be provided. For proper bone growth, calcium and phosphorous are necessary in a ratio of 1-2 parts calcium to 1 part phosphorous. Bone meal and dicalcium phosphate are excellent sources of calcium and phosphorous. Limestone provides calcium but no phosphorous. In certain areas, trace minerals such as zinc, copper, molybdenum, potassium, and selenium are deficient in the soil and need to be supplemented in the feed.

To complete the many complex functions in the body, vitamins are necessary. In the growing animal, the essential vitamins are provided in the milk. As the animal matures, most of the vitamins needed can be produced in the digestive tract. Vitamin A and E are provided by green forages, and sunlight provides a usable form of vitamin D. If there is a shortage of vitamins, they must be provided in the feed or given by an injection.

RATION FORMULATION

A ration that meets all the needs of an animal is said to be balanced. It will provide the energy, protein, minerals, vitamins, and water in sufficient quantities to meet the needs of an animal for body maintenance, growth, reproduction, and lactation. In simple terms, a balanced daily ration is one which provides an animal the proper proportions and amounts of nutrients for a period of 24 hours.

In formulating a ration, feeds are placed in three different groups: (1) roughage, (2) concentrates, (3) vitamin and mineral supplements.

Roughages are very important in all ruminants to maintain a healthy intestinal system as well as providing nutrients. There should be a balance of fiber, non-fiber energy source, digestible protein, and fat to achieve the maximum production or function.

Concentrates supply most of the protein and energy in a ration. In high producing animals, most of the dry matter intake will come from this source. In considering the digestibility of concentrates, attention should be given to the physical form of the feed materials; the maturity at harvest time and how long it has been stored.

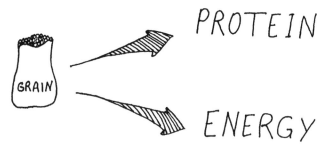

Grain provides protein and energy.

In balancing a ration, supplements are considered once the protein and energy levels have been met. When deficiencies are found, they are added either as a mixture, or fed separately. These supplements are usually referred to as the micro-nutrients.

Some major points should be considered when formulating a ration. These include:

1. Availability and cost of the feed ingredients.
2. Moisture content. This is more important in the case of high moisture grain or silage.
3. Composition of the feeds. Use book values as guides only.
4. Quality of feed.
5. Degree of processing of the feed.
6. Soil analysis where the feeds originated.
7. Nutrient requirements for the animals involved.

The nutrient requirements will depend on production goals, and will vary according to size, age, sex, growth rate, reproductive state, and work expected.

Before feed can be evaluated for its nutritional value, it should be converted to a 100% dry matter basis. This becomes especially important when feeding high moisture feeds such as silage or fresh legumes. When the moisture content is known, conversion tables can be used to determine the percent dry matter.

A laboratory analysis of the available feeds is the most accurate way to know what their nutrient contents are. If this is not possible or is impractical, we can use feed-composition tables to give us a close idea of what the nutritive values are. These values will vary according to maturity at harvest, moisture, soil climate, and storage conditions.

Local agriculture extension agencies should be contacted for assistance in determining these values.

Raising cattle in the tropics can present special problems with nutrition. Tropical forages mature quicker than those in temperate zones. As a result they have lower levels of protein, minerals, energy, and higher levels of crude fiber. Digestion of forages which are high in crude fiber slow the digestive tract resulting in less total food consumption. Tropical forages also have a higher water content which reduces the energy intake. Some steps which can be taken to reduce these problems are:

1. Cutting grasses for green chop in the morning.
2. Allowing the grass to wilt in the sunshine.
3. Feeding the dried feed in the evening or the next day.

The two most common ways to balance rations for cattle are the square (Pearson Square) method and the trial and error method. With the introduction of computer technology, many programs have been written to facilitate ration formulation.

By using the Pearson Square method, one has a simple, direct and easy way to calculate proportions between two ingredients. Quick substitutions of feed can be made in keeping with market fluctuations without disturbing the protein content. When using this method, it is recognized that one specific nutrient alone receives major consideration. In other words, it is a method of balancing one nutrient requirement without consideration of the other nutrients.

To balance rations by the square method, or by any other method, it is first necessary to have available the nutrient requirements and feed composition tables. The following is an example of how the square method is used in formulating a ration:

Example. A dairy farmer has a 300 kg cow that is in the middle of her lactation. He would like to feed her a ration containing 16% protein and has available Coastal Bermuda grass hay which is 10.5% protein and corn containing 8.9% protein. What percent of the ration should consist of corn and Bermuda grass?

The procedure for balancing this ration is as follows:

1. Draw a square, and place the number 16 (desired protein) in the center.
2. At the upper left-hand corner of the square, write Bermuda grass and its protein content (10.5); at the lower lefthand corner, write corn and its protein content (8.9).
3. Subtract diagonally across the square (the smaller number from the larger), and record the difference at the corners on the right-hand side (16 - 10.5 = 5.5; 16 - 8.9 = 7.1). The number at the

upper right-hand corner gives the parts of Bermudagrass by weight, and the number at the lower right-hand corner gives the parts of corn by weight to balance a ration with 16% protein.

Bermuda grass	10.5		7.1 Parts Corn
		16	
Corn	8.9		5.5 Parts Bermuda grass
			12.6 Total parts

4. To determine what percent of the ration would be Bermuda grass, divide the parts of Bermuda grass by the total parts and multiply by 100 (example: 7.1 / 12.6 X 100 = 56%). The remainder, 44%, would be corn.

Another method involves simple mathematics in a step wise manner of using the available feed and calculating how it will meet the requirements of the animal. To illustrate this method, we will balance a ration for a 400kg cow, not giving milk, in a penned area in the middle third of her pregnancy.

First we will need to identify what feeds are available and determine their composition. In this case let's assume we have a small field of molasses grass which is cut by hand daily after growing for about 50 days. Also available is a smaller plot of sugarcane molasses. We know the nutrient content of these two feeds to be:

	% DM	% TDN	Mcal/ kg ME	% CP	% Ca	% P
Molasses grass (50 days' growth)	22	53	1.9	9.0	.63	.54
Sugarcane molasses	77	53	1.92	5.4	1.09	.12

Note: Mcal/ is one million calories
DM is the Dry Matter.
TDN is the Total Digestible Nutrients.
ME is the Metabolizable Energy.
CP is Crude Protein.
Ca is Calcium.
P is Phosphorus.

Since the animal can only eat a limited amount of dry matter, this becomes the deciding factor in the ration. Generally animals eat *2-3% of their body weight daily* if they are producing milk or carrying a calf. It should be remembered that the natural or wet form of the feed weighs more than when dry. In this case with the molasses grass having a

22% dry matter, the wet form would weigh 78% more. The TDN and ME are calculated on a dry matter basis. Since Ca and P are essential nutrients, they are also listed and should be balanced in the final ration. Next, we need to find the animal's requirements. From available tables, we know approximately what she needs on a daily basis according to her size and state of pregnancy.

Animal class	kg DM	kg TDN	Mcal ME	gm CP	gm Ca	gm P
Cow, 400kg, middle third of pregnancy	7.5	3.6	13.1	525	13	13

Since molasses grass is the most abundant feed, it should be considered first. From the above chart we see that the cow will eat about 7.5 kg\day of dry matter. If we multiply the values from the composition table of molasses grass by 7.5, we see what nutrients are provided by eating only this forage. The following values found are:

	kg DM	kg TDN	Mcal ME	gm CP	gm Ca	gm P
Molasses grass forage provides	7.5	3.97	14.25	675	47.25	40.5

Now we can evaluate the diet. We really have more than enough of each nutrient for the cow, and no other feed is necessary to meet the daily needs. Since there is an oversupply of most of the nutrients, we could reduce the amount of feed somewhat and still meet the requirements.

The diet should now be converted from dry matter to a wet, as fed basis. To determine the amount to be fed each day of the molasses grass, we divide the amount of dry matter eaten each day (7.5kg) by the dry matter content of the molasses grass (22%). We then see that the cow will have to eat 34.9kg/ day of the fresh forage (7.5kg / 22% = 34.9kg). In many cases, it is not possible for the animal to eat the amount of fresh food necessary to meet all the requirement. Consideration should be made to dry or wilt the forage before feeding or to add a higher energy supplement.

In summary, what we need to balance a ration for livestock is:

1. An idea of the nutritional requirements.
2. A list of the feeds available.
3. The composition of the feeds.

Make the calculations on a dry matter basis and evaluate the results by comparing the requirements with the compositions of the feeds. Make any adjustments needed, then convert from a dry matter to an as fed basis adding supplements such as concentrates if necessary.

To complete the ration formulation, supplements are generally considered after the macro-nutrients (protein and energy) have been balanced. The most common mineral we need to remember is salt (sodium chloride). It is necessary for body cells to function, in addition to being an appetite stimulator. Either block of loose salt should be available to cattle at all times. The average mature cow should have 40-50 gm/per day. Trace minerals are also needed in small amounts for proper health. Plants contain minerals but there may not be enough to meet the requirements. In tropical areas, the mineral content of plants may be less than in temperate climates. Deficiencies of minerals may result in loss of condition, patchy bald areas, abortion, diarrhea, anemia, loss of appetite, and a craving for dirt or wood. If possible, the trace minerals should be provided in a loose form for free choice consumption.

The amount and kind of minerals to supplement will vary as to the climate and soil conditions. Calcium and phosphorous are the two most common minerals that may be deficient.

Table 4: Suggested Mineral Requirements (Dry Basis).

	Beef cattle	Lactating dairy cows
Macroelements		
calcium (%)	.28	.52
phosphorus (%)	.25	.36
magnesium (%)	.1	.2
potassium (%)	.65	.8
sodium (%)	.08	.18
sulfur (%)	.1	.2
Microelements		
cobait (ppm)	.1	.1
copper (ppm)	8.0	10.0
iodine (ppm)	.5	.5
iron (ppm)	50.0	50.0
manganese (ppm)	40.0	40.0
molybdenum (ppm)	--	--
selenium (ppm)	.2	.1
zinc (ppm)	30.0	40.0

Adapted from McDowell (1985). Note: The true requirements will range higher and lower because of various dietary and animal factors.

To provide the animal easy access to the minerals, they are often mixed with salt. To encourage consumption, the mixtures should be placed in areas where the cattle tend to congregate or at watering facilities.

Vitamins are also found in most plant materials, but like minerals, they may need to be supplemented. They are necessary for many functions in the body and should not be overlooked in the overall ration. Vitamin A is the one vitamin that is often supplemented in the feed or by injection. This vitamin becomes more important if the animal is not consuming fresh, green feed or legumes. Other vitamins such as D, E, K, B, and C may need to be added in small amounts.

FORAGE PRODUCTION AND UTILIZATION

If one is to realize the maximum production from livestock, one must provide them with the best forage available. Just as selecting a bull with superior offspring and a cow with high yields of milk for a breeding program, the forage should also be genetically superior.

Since a farmer's livestock is his principal source of wealth, security, and pride, one must bring together the knowledge of nutrition, animal health, and management to have a successful operation that will have lasting benefits. Without effective forage to provide nutrition, a strong livestock program cannot be realized.

Before attempting to set up a plan for growing forage, one must be sure that the two least expensive, but most important products are available, water and minerals. An average cow may need up to 12 gallons (48 liters) of water a day for maintenance and production. Salt and trace minerals are also necessary. To assure adequate intake, two feeding locations should be available. In one place, just plain salt, and in the other, a 1:1 mix of dicalcium phosphate and trace mineral salt.

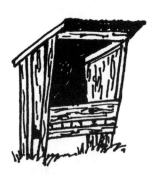

Box of salt and box of salt mixture (1:1 dicalcium phosphate and trace mineral salt)

Mineral Feeder

Since concentrates are usually expensive and in short supply, the goal should be to produce meat and milk from forages alone; except for water, salt, vitamin, and mineral supplements.

To plan for an effective forage program, one needs to know how many livestock can be fed from the available land. Considerations to be made depend on the age and size of the cattle, the rainfall, and the type of pasture available.

One cow can be supported on 0.5 hectares in the tropics, but in drier areas as much as 10 hectares may be needed. Cattle over one year of age will need twice as much forage as younger cattle. A soil test is a good idea before deciding what improvements should be made. Without the results of a test, one can only guess what nutrients need to be added to the soil to obtain the maximum production. The ph or acid/base relationship should also be determined to see if lime needs to be added. Depending on the testing results, nitrogen, phosphorous, potassium, sulphur and other nutrients may need to be added to provide the correct balance.

When animal manure is used to fertilize the ground, there may be a deficiency of phosphorus as this mineral is low in animal waste. The response of plants to fertilizers is in relation to the element found in the least amount, therefore, supplementing with phosphorus when using manure will allow greater utilization of the nitrogen and potassium present.

Weeds are described as a plant growing out of place or a plant that does not contribute to the production of meat or milk. To have a productive pasture, weeds must be controlled. The most common way to do this is by manual removal, herbicides, fertilizers, clipping, or by the use of goats, or a combination of these methods.

HAY PRODUCTION

In order to provide feed for the cattle during periods when fresh pasture is not available, it is necessary to produce hay from surplus feed during the growing season. By doing this a steady supply of nutritious feed can be available throughout the year. Simply stated, hay production is the process of cutting fresh grasses and legumes during the growing season, followed by drying and storing the resulting product.

To assure the highest nutritional level, it is important to cut the forage just before the plant flowers. If it is allowed to mature, the yield and quality of the hay is decreased. In addition, cattle will not have a very good appetite for hay that is too mature.

It is best to wait until the morning dew has evaporated from the grass before cutting it. The cut forage should lay on the ground to dry for at least one to three days before gathering it. Try to avoid letting the hay get wet from rain or from drying too much. Important nutrients are lost if the hay is not harvested soon after being cut.

At the proper time, small piles can be gathered with a rack or fork and hauled to an accessible area for feeding, and made into larger stacks of up to 10 meters. It should be in a dry, well drained area and a fence should be present to keep cattle away. Each stack should peak in the center or be covered to keep the rain from running into the center.

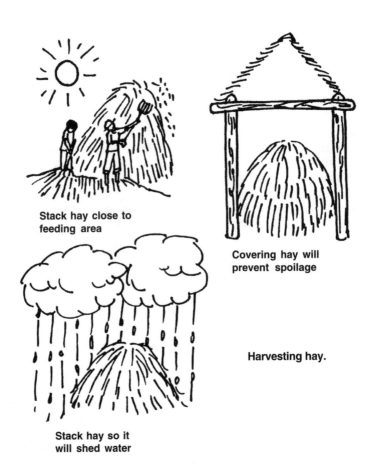

Stack hay close to feeding area

Covering hay will prevent spoilage

Harvesting hay.

Stack hay so it will shed water

Another way to preserve forages is to turn the freshly cut plant into silage. Some of the more common feeds used for silage are rapid growing plants such as corn, sorghum, and grasses. Instead of allowing the cut material to dry, it is placed in a special pit or upright silo where it undergoes fermentation which protects the nutrients in the plants. This type of storage takes special planning and preparation to avoid loss from spoilage. Although silage has certain advantages, it is also more difficult to produce. Conditions such as the moisture content of the feed, the temperature, and the fermentation process are very important in silage production. It should be attempted only after careful study.

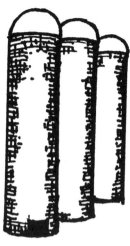

Upright Silo

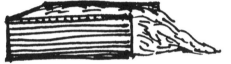

Trench or horizontal silo

Section IV

Reproduction

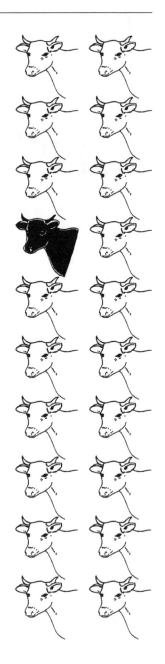

BREEDING MANAGEMENT

In any breeding program the goal should be to increase the productivity of the offspring. In cattle we are interested primarily with meat and milk production, but other traits such as birth weight, weaning weight, disease resistance, and carcass qualities are also important.

Most breeding programs are concerned with using the most rapid method of improving the genetics of the offspring. This usually involves bringing into the herd exotic breeds especially those of European ancestry. The biggest problem with this method is the death loss from disease and lack of adaptation to the local management practices. The ability to resist local diseases and survive is necessary for a breeding program to be successful.

One alternative to using exotic breeds for improving milk and meat production is to use a selection process with the native animal population. Although this process takes much longer to register improvement compared to the introduction of exotic breeds, it may be more economical and more practical due to the high death and production losses of the exotics.

This system would have to involve an animal identification system, controlled or selective breeding, and a record of events. A commitment of individuals and organizations would be required to obtain the desired results. This may take ten years or longer to select families of cattle with greater potential than their herd mates.

In the selection of a bull, careful attention should be given to the characteristics of his offspring and his parents. Traits to select for include milk production, birth weight, weaning weight, yearling weight, carcass weight and disease resistance. It is important to remember that the bull contributes 50% of the genetic to the offspring and that his daughters will go on to become replacement females. Because of this relationship, it is estimated that the bull can contribute up to 80 % of the genetic material in a herd over a period of time.

In some herds, inbreeding (mating of related animals) is practiced. This is generally not recommended because of the increase of the undesirable traits of the parents. Some of the traits that may be seen are early death, stunted offspring, dwarfism, hydrocephalus (water on the brain), deformed joints, and nervous disorders. Cleft palate (open area in roof of the mouth), curved spine, stiff joints, and double muscling are other signs of inbreeding. It is a practice to avoid if possible.

SELECTION OF THE BULL

Traits to look for in selecting a bull are proper conformation and general appearance. The feet and legs should be sound. Testicle size is also important as improved fertility is generally related to this trait. The

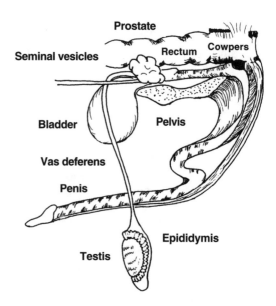

Reproductive organs of the bull.

Prostate

Seminal vesicles

Rectum　Cowpers

Bladder　Pelvis

Vas deferens

Penis

Epididymis

Testis

ability of the bull to pass on his traits to his offspring is very important in the breeding program.

The reproductive organs are shown in figure 1. The sperm is produced in the testicles and stored in the seminal vesicles until ejaculation. Several factors can affect the quality and quantity of semen including environmental temperatures, sickness, or local infections. If possible, semen should be collected by a trained person and evaluated for reproductive ability.

SELECTION OF THE FEMALE

Many traits should be considered when selecting a female. Since meat and milk production is one of the most important factors we are looking for, it would be given priority. There are many other considerations however, such as fertility or reproduction ability, conformation, disease resistance, and ease of handling or temperament. It may be desirable to choose a breed that suits the management style of an individual or farm. This is especially important when there is a shortage of labor and facilities to work the cattle. Certain breeds are noted for their gentle temperament and may be better for small operations.

REPRODUCTION

In the natural breeding process with a bull, the female is only receptive during a certain time period called "heat' or estrus. If the cow is in good health and receiving adequate nutrition, she will cycle through an estrus period every 21 days. The estrus lasts approximately 18 hours, and she will ovulate or release an egg about 11 hours after the end of the estrus period. Since the egg is released after the "heat" period, it is best to expose the bull to the cow towards the end of the estrus rather than at the beginning. It is very important that the cow be at a high level of nutrition when attempting to breed her. In fact she should be gaining weight at the time of breeding.

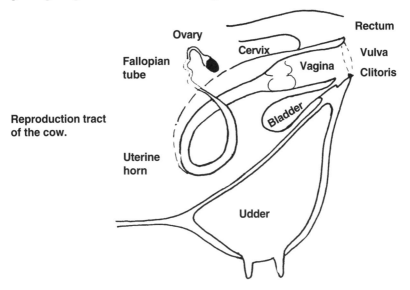

Reproduction tract of the cow.

The most common signs of estrus are bellowing, restlessness, mounting of other cows or standing while other cows mount her. A slight discharge of mucous is often seen coming from the vagina and the cow will be attracted to the bull.

As mating takes place, the bull deposits his ejaculate in the vagina. Thousands of sperm enter the vagina with the breeding act. Some of the sperm cells pass through the cervix and into the uterus. It is in the fallopian tube that fertilization takes place by only one sperm cell. The fertilized egg then travels into the uterus and attaches to the uterine body. The developing fetus becomes enclosed in a sack called the placenta. Nutrition is supplied through the umbilical cord by the transfer of nutrients from the mother's blood.

Before breeding the cow, it is important that she is of proper size and weight. Although this will vary with breeds, in general she should be at least 18 months of age and be in a rapid weight gaining stage. Females will start the estrus cycle as early as six months of age but are not ready for breeding at that time. When a cow has delivered a calf, she should have a minimum of 2 months rest before re-breeding.

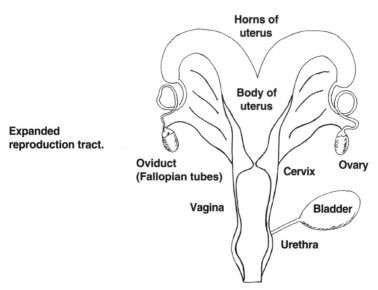

Horns of uterus

Body of uterus

Expanded reproduction tract.

Oviduct (Fallopian tubes)

Cervix

Ovary

Vagina

Bladder

Urethra

This allows the uterus to clean itself and for the cow to regain her nutritional status.

If possible the cow should be examined to determine if she is pregnant after breeding. This is most commonly done 60 days after exposure to the bull. An experienced person can feel the developing fetus through rectal palpation. It is important to determine pregnancy, as an infection of the uterus can cause the cow to not show signs of estrus as well. It also avoids feeding and caring for a cow which may not be pregnant.

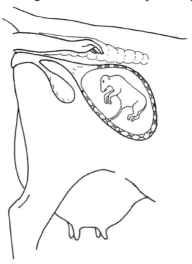

Rectal palpation of the fetus.

Section V

Artificial Insemination

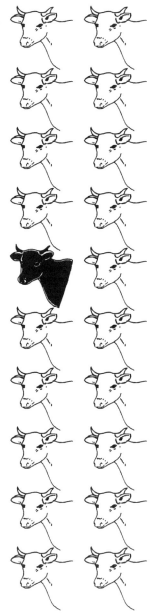

ARTIFICIAL INSEMINATION IN CATTLE

Beginning in the late 1940's, the introduction of artificial insemination (AI) in the more developed countries of the world, has exerted a very positive influence in the beef and dairy cattle industry. When original stock are bred with improved semen, the offspring will produce substantially more milk and meat. In addition, AI has provided a practical solution for the control of infectious diseases which affect the reproductive tract.

Ideally, AI makes it possible for the most humble cattle owner to obtain calves from valuable bulls. The possession of offspring from "great" bulls can provide owners with the incentive to improve the overall practices of feeding, management, and disease control in their herd.

In recognizing the importance of cattle for improving the economic level of families in underdeveloped communities, it seems reasonable to include AI in the planning of new development programs. Raising the "genetic ceiling" can be a direct route toward a better livestock economy.

Technically, one may think of AI as a series of controlled steps which can be simplified to include:

(1) Collection of semen from a quality bull
(2) Depositing the semen in the reproductive tract of a female cow.

For AI, a device called an artificial vagina is used to collect semen from a bull by either natural or stimulated methods.

Drawing of an artificial vagina.

Water Intake

Warm water

Rubber tunnel

Artificial vagina (birth canal)

Test tube

46

The semen is first examined with the aid of a microscope to be sure it is normal. It is then combined with materials that provide protection and nourishment. These also "extend" the semen without loss of fertility, thereby making possible insemination of many cows from a single collection. The few bulls needed in AI can be maintained under close veterinary supervision, assuring consistent high fertility of their semen and freedom from infectious diseases.

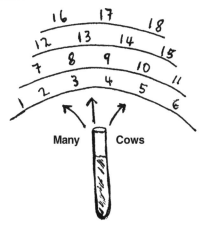

Example of one vial of semen used to breed many cows.

Many　　Cows

Semen

In the very early days of AI, semen kept at 34 to 38 degrees F (2-4 degrees C) was usable for only a few days. However, since the late 1950's, most semen is preserved by a special freezing process and stored in liquid nitrogen at -320 degrees F (-195 degrees C). Frozen semen not only has the advantage of being preserved indefinitely, but, may be transported and stored for use at almost any location in the world.

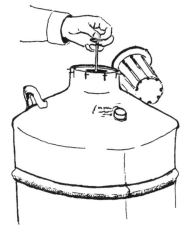

Insemination tanks and semen holders

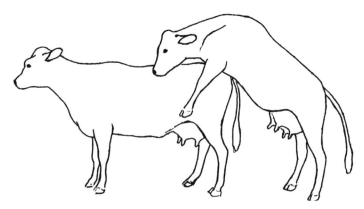

A cow mounting another cow.

Females are only fertile at the time of ovulation or during their "heat" period. This occurs in mature, healthy heifers and non pregnant cows approximately every three weeks. Estrus or "heat" is recognized by certain signs, such as restlessness, bawling, and an enlargement of the vulva. The most critical sign of estrus is standing and accepting being mounted by a bull or another female. Late in estrus, an egg cell is released from an ovary. Union of one sperm and one egg mark the beginning of pregnancy.

A well trained inseminator/technician can instruct cattle owners on how to recognize the signs of estrus. When heifers of cows are ready to breed, the inseminator/technician must be advised promptly.

The inseminator/technician will thaw a unit of frozen semen. Next, working with one hand in the rectum for control of the female organ, the inseminator/technician will insert a tubular instrument used to deposit semen in the proper location.

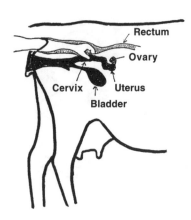

Hand in the rectumholding the cervix.

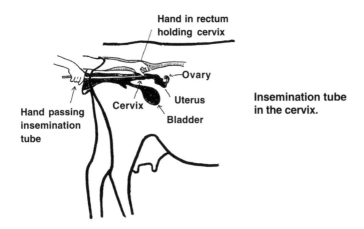

Hand in rectum holding cervix

Ovary

Uterus

Cervix

Bladder

Hand passing insemination tube

Insemination tube in the cervix.

The probability of a successful pregnancy varies from 50% to 70% at each insemination.

Heifers and cows intended to be inseminated must be kept separate at all times from a bull to avoid a natural breeding. If necessary, fencing or castration of other bulls on the farm may become necessary. Restraint of heifers and cows while awaiting or during insemination can vary from use of a rope to a very simple breeding chute.

PLANNING AN AI PROGRAM

Serious consideration and long range planning must precede any AI program. Experience has shown that to be successful and to achieve permanent values, an AI program must be a long term commitment. Improved husbandry practices such as proper nutrition, disease control, and management must be part of the overall program.

At least three to three and a half years are required before the first generation of AI heifers can be milked. This includes nine months of pregnancy for a mother cow, 18 to 24 months for a heifer to mature, then nine months of pregnancy before she will deliver a calf.

There is no reason for a new AI service to be concerned with producing its own semen. Worthy bulls, trained laboratory workers, and equipment are usually expensive and unavailable locally. Rather, it is better to concentrate all local resources and efforts on the single goal of getting as many superior calves as possible from the existing heifers and cows.

There are many well established and reliable organizations in the business of producing and marketing bull semen. Bulls of different levels of merit and breeds are available. This means that high quality semen is available at relatively low cost from superior bulls that are well suited genetically for use in a beginning AI service.

49

Serious thought must be given to the choice of the new breed/breeds of cattle to be introduced. Under the stressful environmental conditions of the tropics, there is a limit to the percent of modern, temperate climate "blood" (Bos taurus) that can be tolerated. First cross offspring of Holstein, Brown Swiss, and Jersey usually do well. Both beef and milking strains of humped cattle (Bos indicus) (Zebu, Brahman) are available from the USA.

It is especially important that arrangements be made with a semen supplier willing and able to provide more than just semen. There will be a need for:

1) Buying or renting the right kind of equipment for local storage and transport.
2) Periodic, reliable, resupply of liquid nitrogen.
3) Training and support of a competent inseminator/technician.
4) Necessary inseminating supplies.
5) Timely experienced advice and counsel.

Experience has shown that a well trained, competent, and conscientious inseminator/technician is the key to success. Cattle owners must be taught their responsibilities and continuously encouraged. On a day by day basis this is an ongoing job for the AI technician.

As mentioned earlier, it is essential that heifers and cows intended to be inseminated be kept separate from bulls. The means to accomplish this may challenge local practices and traditions. Never-the-less, separation must be accomplished!

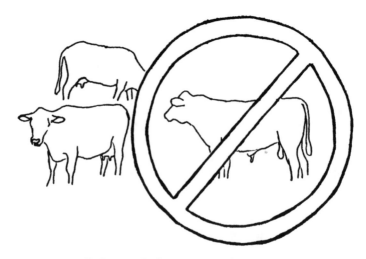

Bulls must be kept separate from cows.

In some communities, heifers and cows have by custom been taken to bulls for breeding, and recognition of the signs of heat may already be well understood. In other cases it needs to be taught. With experience, many individuals become very proficient in recognizing when their cow is ready to breed.

Obviously, the inseminator must be available when heifers and cows are ready for breeding. This means availability seven days a week. Reliable transportation is very important for transport of the frozen semen, for insemination equipment, and for the AI technician. For transport; autos, motorbikes, bicycles, horses, mules and other animals are often used in various parts of the world.

In order to minimize travel, it is often necessary to develop some system of communication to advise the AI technician when he/she is needed. Many ingenious methods have been used, reflecting local circumstances.

The cost of a calf from an AI program will be largely determined by the total number of heifers and cows inseminated in a given period of time. Until the number of successful inseminations are quite high, the fixed costs of the program (equipment, refrigerant, transportation for semen and AI technician, salary for the inseminator, etc.) will be the greater part of the cost of each calf born from AI.

An AI program must be designed to fit its local conditions as no two communities are the same. Inseminations must be made when the heifers and cows are ready, not when "we" are ready. In some locations the time for breeding may be distinctly seasonal, and AI programs may be planned to operate only certain months of the year.

If the conditions can come together to meet the above requirements, farmers can realize a great improvement in their local livestock by using AI programs. It follows that economic gain should result benefiting both individual families and communities.

Section VI

Calving

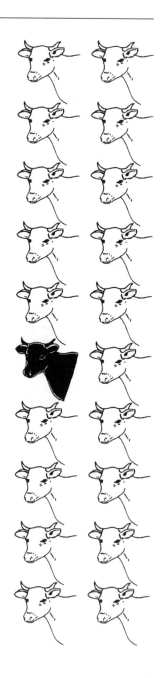

CARE OF THE COW BEFORE AND DURING CALVING

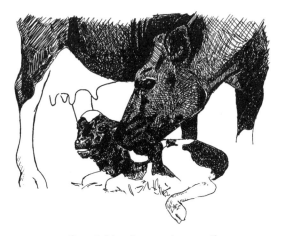

Cow licking her newborn calf.

As the time approaches for a cow is to deliver her calf, she must be observed very carefully. A clean, grassy area is an excellent birthing bed in a mild, dry climate. If the weather is wet, rainy or cold, a clean dry pen of suitable construction should be provided. A plan to restrict the cow's movement if assistance needs to be given is very important. This could be something as simple as a rope with a secure holding point or a pen or barn for confinement.

As calving time nears, several signs may be noted. Among these are a relaxing of the ligaments around the tail head and pelvis, enlargement of the vulva, and a mucus discharge from the reproductive tract. These signs will be evident about 24 to 72 hours before calving. The udder becomes distended and may begin to drip milk as the time for calving approaches. A swelling (edema) may develop under the stomach just before the cow goes into labor. A more imminent sign of calving is elevation of the tail and straining periodically.

As true labor approaches, the cow will generally lie down and show strong contractions. The "water-bag" appearing is the first sign that the cervix is open and that actual calving has begun. From this point, it should be less than two hours for the calf to Be born. If hard labor begins and no calf is delivered within two hours, the cow should be examined to determine if there is a problem, and assistance given as necessary.

Most cows will deliver their calf with little or no difficulty. However, situations arise when the cow requires assistance. Sometimes these problems are easily corrected and rather simple, other times great dexterity and strength may be required to manipulate the calf for the correct presentation. In some cases, such as the presence of milk fever or parturient paresis, the calving problem is a disease problem that needs treatment before or while the calf is being delivered.

When examining the cow, the examiner should be as clean as possible. Many diseases that affect the reproductive tract of the cow are transmissible to humans. If possible, protective gloves and clothing should be worn. When protective gear is not available, the operator should use warm water and soap to clean his hands and arms both before, during, and following the delivery to avoid contamination of himself and the cow.

In addition to warm water and soap, other necessary items to have on hand when assisting in calving are obstetrical (OB) chains or ropes, OB handles, and a suitable traction system such as a calf puller. In the absence of traction devices, additional people should be available to assist the operator.

The normal presentation of a calf for delivery is front feet first with the head extended on top of the legs with the nose at the knees (Fig. 1). This is called anterior presentation.

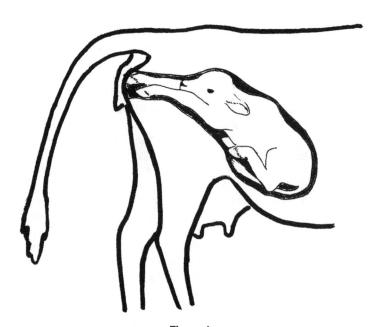

Figure 1.

With this presentation, one difficulty that can arise is the calf may be too large to pass through the pelvis of the cow. If the examiner can pass a hand between the top of the calf's head and the pelvis of the cow, generally the calf can be delivered with slight traction. If there is no space available, a caesarian section (operation) or a fetotomy (cutting the calf in small pieces) must be considered. In a fetotomy, the fetus is removed in small sections using a special cutting wire to avoid injury to the cow. These procedures should only be done by a skilled and experienced person, preferably a veterinarian.

The most common problem associated with anterior presentation is that one or both of the front legs may be folded back. When the cow is examined, the head is in the pelvis with one or both legs absent from view.

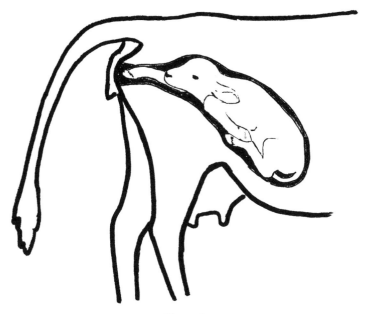

Figure 2.

In this case (Fig. 2), the head must be forced back, so that the operator may reach the leg or legs that are folded back. When there is enough room to locate the leg, the knee joint (the second joint up from the hoof) needs to be identified. This joint has to be forced upward. As the leg is brought up, generally a chain or rope can be looped around the leg and forced downward until the loop is located between the fetlock (the first joint up from the hoof) and the hoof.

With one hand moving the knee up and back, gentle and firm traction is applied to the chain by the other hand until the lower leg is brought into the birth canal and extended into the pelvis. Extreme care must be taken to protect the uterus and vagina from the sharp hoof as it is rotated upwards. This is best done by placing a hand over the tip of the hoof as it is pulled into the pelvis. If both legs are absent from the pelvis, the procedure is repeated for the second leg. In some cases it is impossible to push the head back to get at the legs. Then it is necessary to amputate the head to allow room to manipulate the legs as described above.

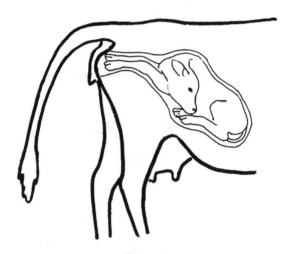

Figure 3.

When there is an anterior presentation, but with the head turned back, (Fig. 3) the legs need to be forced back in. The head is then located and pulled into the pelvis. When the head is securely in the pelvis, the legs can be brought to normal position and the calf delivered.

Posterior presentation (Fig. 4) is when the calf is presented with the back legs and tail coming into the pelvis.

The most common problem with this presentation is failure of the calf to be delivered quickly enough to insure its survival. Once the umbilical cord is broken, the calf attempts to breathe and inhales fetal fluids. The lungs fill with fluid and the calf drowns. When this condition is diagnosed, the calf should be pulled quickly to increase the chances of survival. Time is of the essence!

Often with posterior presentation, both back legs are folded forward and only the tail is in the pelvis (Fig. 5). The tail may be presented through the vagina in some cases of prolonged labor.

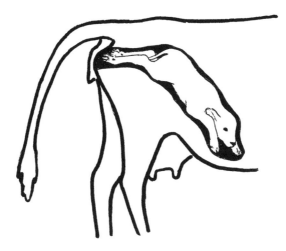

Figure 4.

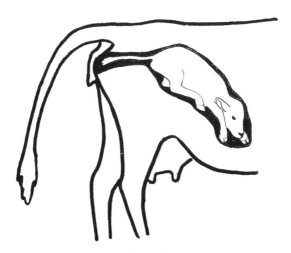

Figure 5.

To correct this presentation, pressure must be applied to the calf's pelvis to push it forward. The hock joint is then brought up to the brim of the pelvis. This is repeated for the second leg. When both hocks are on the brim of the pelvis, a chain needs to be attached between the fetlocks and the hoof. Steady traction is applied to the chain as the hock is pushed forward, upward, and to the side. Here again the hoof should be protected so that it does not injure the uterus or vagina as it

57

is extracted. When the first leg has been extended, the process is repeated with the second leg. The calf can then be delivered. Many times when this presentation is found, the cow has twins and should be checked first for a second calf.

Sometimes a calf will be "upside down" (Fig. 6). When this position is observed, it needs to be determined if the calf is actually in the wrong position or if there is a torsion or twisting of the vagina and uterus. Careful, gentle, slow entry of the hand into the vagina will allow detection of a torsion.

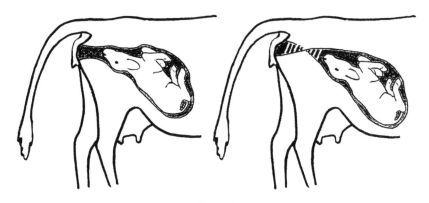

Figure 6.

Most often a fold or ridge can be felt in the birth canal that curves up and around. The torsion can either be clockwise or counter clockwise although most are counter clockwise. It is best to try to correct the twist manually by rotating the calf into normal position before trying to bring the feet into the birth canal. This is a difficult task and requires strong arms. To accomplish the rotation a hand is introduced alongside the calf and an attempt is made to roll the calf in the opposite direction of the twist. Getting the calf to rock back and forth and then giving one hard push will often correct the torsion. Some torsions cannot be reduced in this way. Another technique can be used if there are several people to help. The cow is cast using a rope. She is made to lie on the same side as the direction of the twist (most commonly on the left). Using ropes tied to her feet, the cow is rolled in the direction of the twist. She is then allowed to get up, and an examination is made to see if the torsion was corrected. The procedure may be repeated if necessary. Many times the calf will have to be delivered by caesarian section when a torsion is present, because the cervix does not dilate enough to allow the calf to pass even though the torsion may be corrected.

If there is no torsion and the calf is upside down, it can be manipulated around by pushing on the head and twisting the legs. Once the calf is in normal position, it can be delivered.

There are variations of the abnormal positions discussed above, but most will fall under the descriptions noted. Assisting in calving can be a difficult and exhausting procedure. If possible, it is best to have an experienced person or veterinarian available to minimize the dangers to both the cow and calf.

Section **VII**

Care of Cow
After Calving

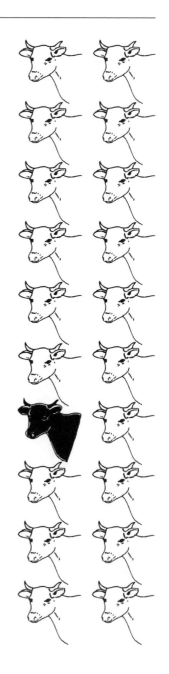

CARE OF THE FRESH COW

There are many problems that can occur to the fresh cow that are directly related to the birth of her calf. Some of these are very serious and life threatening, therefore, careful observation must be given to the cow for the first few days following calving. A uterine (womb) prolapse usually occurs immediately or within 48 hours after the calf is born. It should be treated as an emergency, as the cow can go into shock and die within a short period of time. Occasionally a complication occurs when the cow has milk fever (parturient paresis) at the same time. If this occurs, treatment must be given to correct the milk fever before replacing the prolapsed uterus. After an injection of a spinal anesthesia to relax the straining contractions of the cow, the uterus is washed with clean water and soap and very carefully replaced back inside the cow. There are many techniques to aid in replacement of the uterus, most of which involve elevating the hindquarters of the cow by various means. If the cow is lying down, this is done by extending the rear legs backwards. Once replacement has been accomplished, the uterus should be returned as much as possible in its original position by pushing gently with a closed fist into each uterine horn. Following this, the vulva should be sutured and antibiotics administered for 4-5 days to prevent infection. To aid in the uterus returning to normal size, an injection of oxytocin is often recommended. See illustration:

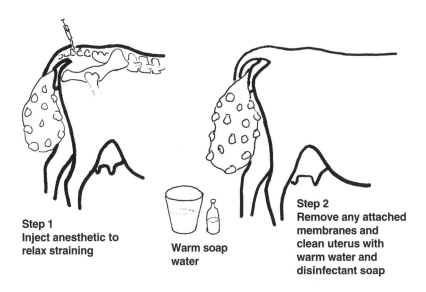

Step 1
Inject anesthetic to
relax straining

Warm soap
water

Step 2
Remove any attached
membranes and
clean uterus with
warm water and
disinfectant soap

61

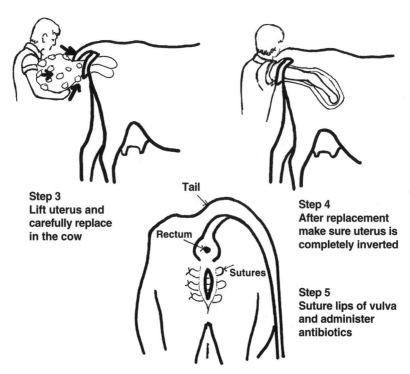

Step 3
Lift uterus and
carefully replace
in the cow

Tail

Rectum

Sutures

Step 4
After replacement
make sure uterus is
completely inverted

Step 5
Suture lips of vulva
and administer
antibiotics

A uterine prolapse and the steps for correction.

RETAINED PLACENTA

When the placenta remains attached in the uterus longer than 24 hours, the cow should be watched closely for signs of infection. In most cases, if the cow does not appear to be sick and is eating well, it is best to let the placenta drop out on its own. This may take up to 10 days. Antibiotics may be given either by injection or into the uterus if deemed necessary. If a decision is made to manually remove the placenta, clean and lubricate the vulva, and use a gloved hand. Careful traction should be used to remove the placental attachments and antibiotics should be administered into the uterus following the procedure.

METRITIS

A condition known as metritis (infection of the uterus) can occur following calving. This is a bacterial infection of the uterus and may cause a mild to severe reaction in the cow. Antibiotics help combat the disease, along with prostaglandins to increase the muscular tone of

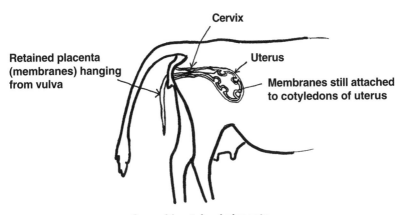

Cervix

Retained placenta (membranes) hanging from vulva

Uterus

Membranes still attached to cotyledons of uterus

Cow with retained placenta.

the uterus. Antibiotics may be given either in the uterus or by injection. Supportive therapy such as oxytocin, antihistamine, and glucose are also used in the treatment.

PYOMETRA

Pyometra (pus in the uterus) is a condition characterized by an accumulation of infected material in the uterus and a retained corpus luteum (yellow body) on an ovary. When this occurs, the cow does not show signs of heat and the owner assumes she is pregnant. A diagnosis is made by rectal palpation and sometimes by observing a yellowish discharge from the vulva. Prostaglandins are the treatment of choice to correct the retained corpus leuteum. They cause the uterus to squeeze out the infected material.

ANESTRUS

A failure to return to heat, or anestrus, is more of a problem when artificial insemination is used. It has been shown that when marker bulls are used, or constant observation is employed 24 hours a day, the cows will be observed in heat. If true anestrus does occur, the feeding program should be examined to check for sufficient energy and protein balance. A blood test to check for anemia may be indicated. In some cases, high milk production may cause anestrus, as well as feet and leg problems.

CYSTIC OVARIES

Cystic ovaries can occur in three different forms, with all affecting the heat cycle.

1. A follicular cyst is the most common form and can cause an anestrus or nymphomania or a very low grade of continuous heat.
2. A failure to ovulate may be the result of a luteal cyst. The cow is usually anestrus because of a production of progesterone which makes the body think it is pregnant.
3. With a cystic corpus luteum, ovulation usually occurs, but sufficient progesterone may not be produced to maintain pregnancy.

The causes of cystic ovaries are related to a lack of the pituitary gland to release sufficient hormones to produce ovulation and the proper development of the ovary. Another cause may be the failure of the hypothalamus (a part of the brain) to produce or release the gonadotropin releasing hormone (GNRH) The treatment for this is an injection of chorionic gonadotropin hormone or gonadotropin releasing hormone. A qualified person familiar with the reproductive system should be consulted when a cow does not show normal heat cycles or fails to get pregnant after two to three breedings.

There are two common metabolic disturbances which occur in cattle associated with calving, ketosis and milk fever.

Ketosis or acetonemia may not occur until a few weeks after the calf is born. It is characterized by low blood sugar which causes loss of appetite, a drop in weight and milk production, and occasionally incoordination. It is caused by not having enough carbohydrates or energy in the diet. The treatment involves correcting the nutritional imbalance. Intravenous injection of glucose, administration of glucocorticoids, and the oral administration of propylene glycol are used to correct the short term symptoms. Ketosis occurs most often in dairy cattle.

Milk fever, or parturient paresis, is an acute condition usually occurring at or soon after calving. The symptoms include a generalized muscle weakness, decreased circulatory output, and coma; leading to death if not treated. It is associated with the sudden onset of milk production in mature cows. The consistent finding is a drop in the calcium level in the blood.

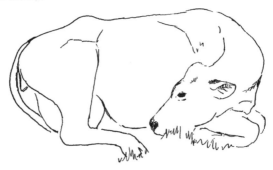

Cow with milk fever

Prevention of this problem usually involves feeding a diet high in phosphorus and low in calcium to stimulate absorption of calcium from skeletal tissue, as well as supplements of vitamin D in the feed before calving. Dosing of calcium in a gel form may also be used just before or after calving to aid in prevention.

The treatment involves the administration of a calcium solution given intravenously, but subcutaneous and intraperitoneal routes can be used. The heart should be monitored carefully during administration of the calcium solution to prevent cardiac arrest. If the beats of the heart become irregular, the rate of giving the calcium should be slowed or stopped until it returns to normal. Occasionally repeat treatments are necessary for complete recovery.

Section VIII

Care of the Newborn

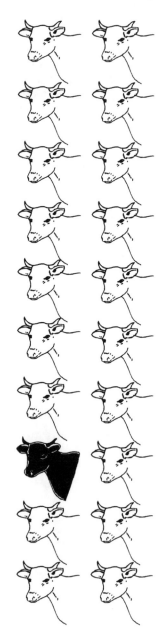

CARE OF THE CALF

As soon as the calf is born, it should be checked for clear air passages and excessive bleeding from the navel. If there appears to be a problem with breathing, the mouth should be checked and cleaned of anything blocking the airway. A common practice is to lift the calf by the rear legs to allow any fluid to drain from the respiratory tract. Breathing can be stimulated by pinching the nose of the calf or by gently inserting a straw in the nose.

The navel should be soaked in a 7% solution of iodine as soon as possible to avoid any bacteria entering the calf's body through the umbilical cord. If there is bleeding, the navel should be tied with a string that has been disinfected with iodine. The tie can be left on, as the cord will normally dry up and fall off in about 10 days.

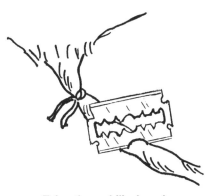

Tying the umbilical cord.

When the calf is breathing normally and is able to sit up, it should be given the cow's "first milk" or colostrum as soon as possible. This is one of the most important steps to aid in the survival and health of the newborn calf. The amount to feed should be approximately 4-5% of the calf's body weight. Since the calf is born with very little resistance to disease and infection, the colostrum is the key to keeping it healthy during the first few weeks of life. True colostrum is defined as the milk obtained from the first milking. Secretions obtained after this for the next 4-5 days are termed transitional milk. Another important fact about colostrum is that the calf loses its ability to absorb the protective substances found in the "first milk" within 24 hours after birth, and that the highest absorption of colostrum occurs within 4 hours after birth. If there is excess colostrum, it can be frozen or allowed to "sour" and fed at a later date to calves as needed.

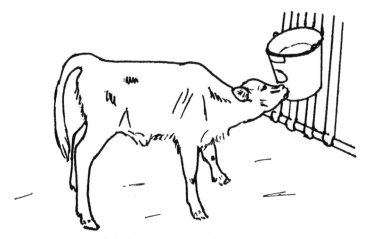

Calf drinking colostrum from a bucket.

When milk production for human consumption is the goal, the calf should be removed from the cow on the first day. For the first two weeks, whole milk should be fed to the calf; after which milk replacers, if available, can be introduced. For calculating the amount of milk to feed, use the formula of 4-5% of the calf's body weight twice daily. If feeding a milk replacer, follow the directions recommended by the manufacturer. When the calf has reached 4-5 weeks of age, grass or a good quality hay should be offered.

If grain is available, it should be introduced in small amounts at 2-4 weeks of age. When the calf is eating 0.5 kilograms (1 pound) per day it can be weaned from the milk or milk replacer. Good quality forage or hay can be fed free choice. The grain can be increased to 2 kilograms (4 pounds) per day, if available, to obtain the optimum growth rate.

Diseases of newborn calves are very significant during the first few weeks of their lives. More young are lost to diarrhea than any other condition. Most problems of diarrhea are related to bacterial, viral, and nutritional causes. Most often a stress such as a change in feeding schedule, movement to new areas, or exposure to bad weather may weaken the calf's resistance. When this happens, organisms that are normally present in the calf but cause no problem, begin to grow rapidly and damage the intestinal tract. The result is diarrhea, where more fluid is lost in the stool than can be taken in by mouth.

Dehydration is the end result which causes death in calves with diarrhea. As fluid is lost, the blood becomes thicker and a condition known as dehydration occurs. The body cannot function when fluids fall below a certain level. Shock follows and results in death unless treated.

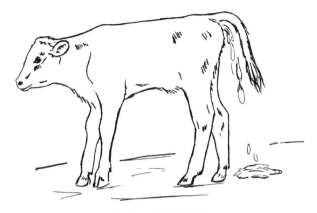

A calf with diarrhea.

To combat the end results of diarrhea and dehydration, treatment should begin as soon as possible with fluids and supportive treatment. Treatment should follow these steps:

Oral fluids.

Replace the nutrients and salts lost through the diarrhea.

Treat with antibiotics. The most common antibiotics used in calf diarrheas are tetracycline, sulfa drugs, and neomycin.

Withhold milk for 24-48 hours. During this time give a milk replacement called oral electrolytes. Either a commercial or a home made solution can be used. A simple mixture can be made by using two litters of water, one tsp. salt, and two tsp of baking soda. From one to two litters should be given two to three times a day until the diarrhea stops. If the calf is to weak to drink, the fluids can be given with a stomach tube.

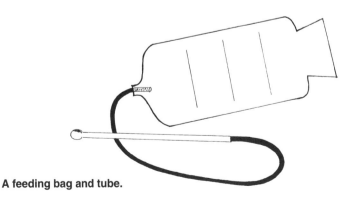

A feeding bag and tube.

Prevention of calf diarrhea or scours is crucial. As mentioned earlier, it is very important to give the newborn the first milk or colostrum within two hours after birth to provide natural protection. Do not allow sick calves to contact healthy ones. Keep the area clean and disinfect equipment between animals. Provide a warm, dry place for the sick calves. Maintain well regulated feeding schedules. Use vaccines if available, to reduce the incidence of infections.

Generally the best way to raise calves is by keeping them in individual pens or hutches. The advantage is that the calf is separated from other calves for disease prevention, and individual care and attention can be given. The disadvantage of this type of housing is the greater expense and labor involved.

The design of the pen should allow a minimum of 1.67 square meters (18 square feet) for calf stalls to 2.22 square meters (24 square feet) for hutches. Hutches should have a fenced in area on the open side of an additional 2.22 square meters (24 square feet). The hutch is framed with 5.08 centimeters by 10.16 centimeters (2 inch by 4 inch) lumber. The sides are 1.21 meters by 2.43 meters (4 feet by 8 feet) and the top is the same dimensions. The back side is 1.21 meters by 1.21 meters (4 feet by 4 feet). The front is left open. The hutch is positioned so that the open side faces the sun. A fence of any material is then constructed in front of the hutch, allowing room for the calf to be outside.

In areas where the cows are housed in stalls or stanchions, the calves can be tied among the cows. While this system is relatively cheap and requires no extra housing, it has the disadvantage of the

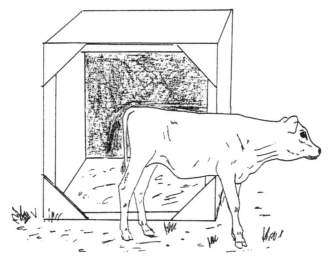

A calf hutch.

70

calves being exposed to the diseases of the cow herd. This should be avoided if possible.

Calves can be individually tied in any area with halters, neck chains or ties. They should be kept at distances such that they cannot suck on each other. A disadvantage of this system is that calves can tangle themselves in their tether and may become injured.

After a calf has been weaned from milk or milk replacer (six to eight weeks of age) and is on a diet of calf starter and grass or hay, it can be grouped with other calves. Generally start with placing three to five animals together, and increase the size of the herd as they grow older. If possible, the calves should be grouped according to size and age. Keep in mind the available space and watering facilities. Overcrowding should be avoided.

After the calves reach one year of age, the numbers are only limited by the facilities available to handle them. From 15 months to two years of age, consideration needs to be given to estrus (heat) detection. For this reason, the animals should be in close proximity so they can be easily observed by the person in charge of the breeding program.

Section IX

Management Tasks

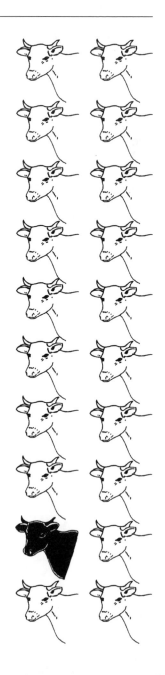

MANAGEMENT TASKS FOR CATTLE

In cattle, there are some important tasks such as castrating, dehorning, and identification, which are much easier and less stressful when done during the first four months of life.

CASTRATION

Any male calves not kept for breeding stock should be castrated as early as possible (from a few days of birth to 3 months). It is much easier to handle very young animals and the side effects of the procedure are minimal during this time. It is a good idea to vaccinate for blackleg and malignant edema to avoid complications following the surgery.

After securing the animal with ropes or with manual restraint, the scrotal area should be cleaned with soap and water and/or a general disinfectant. To prevent infection, the person doing the castration should also have clean hands.

In the technique of "open castration," the bottom one-third of the scrotum is cut off with a sharp knife. The testicles are pulled out of the scrotal sac with steady pressure until the testicular cord breaks. An alternative method is to scrape the cord with a blunt instrument until the cord separates. In young calves there is very little bleeding with this method. Any tissue left hanging from the scrotum should be trimmed with a knife or scissors. Following the operation, a screwworm fly preparation should be applied every 2-3 days until the wound heals. Mild exercise is helpful to avoid swelling.

If the animals are older, the blood supply is greater and care should be taken to avoid bleeding. One way is to tie a knot tightly using a surgical suture (catgut) around the cord. The testicles can then be removed with a knife one to two cm below the suture. Another way to avoid blood loss is to crush the cord and vessels with an instrument called an emasculator.

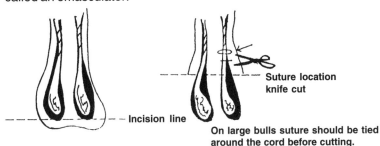

Incision line

Suture location
knife cut

On large bulls suture should be tied
around the cord before cutting.

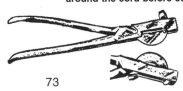

Castration using a suture
and an emasculator.

73

Even when care is taken, bleeding may be a problem when open castration is performed. If there is a steady blood flow for more than 15 minutes, methods should be taken to control blood loss. An absorbent material such as cotton can be packed in the scrotal incision, and the scrotum can be closed with string, sutures, or clothes pins until a blood clot forms. Generally the animal is kept quiet for 12-24 hours and the cotton is removed. An antibiotic such as penicillin should be given and fly repellent applied to prevent screwworm infestation.

There are two methods of "closed castration." One is by placing a special rubber band around the base of the scrotum using a instrument called an elastracator, and the other involves using a procedure of crushing the spermatic cord.

In the rubber band method, the calf is restrained and the band is placed between the testicles and the body wall on the scrotal sac. The blood supply is cut off to the tissue below the rubber band, and after a few days the testicles will shrink and fall off. This type of castration should be used for young animals when the testicles are still small to avoid complications of swelling and infection.

An elastracator with a rubber band attached.

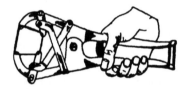

A burdizzo is an instrument which crushes the cord of the testicles without cutting or damaging the scrotum. When this is done correctly, there is no bleeding or danger of infection from screwworms. Once the cord is crushed, the blood supply is cut off and the testicles wither away. It is important that the burdizzo be applied correctly to make sure the cord does not slip sideways from the jaws of the instrument. Each cord should be crushed separately at least twice.

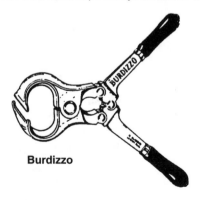

Burdizzo

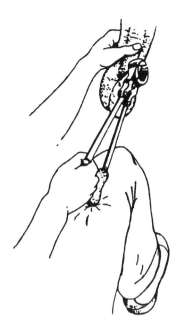

Proper use of a Burdizzo

**A burdizzo being
used for castration.**

DEHORNING

Dehorning is usually performed to keep cattle from injuring humans and each other with their horns. In some areas it is a custom to let the horns grow so the animals will be able to protect themselves from predators.

When dehorning cattle it is desirable to do it as early as possible, before four months of age if convenient. In warm climates, a hot iron is very effective and leaves no blood to attract flies. The iron should be hollowed out to fit around the horn where it can come in contact with the sensitive horn tissue. Usually a few seconds is all that is needed to heat the area around the horns to a desired dark brown color. After a calf is four months of age, the horns are usually too large to remove by this method.

**A hot iron dehorner for calves up to
4-5 months old.**

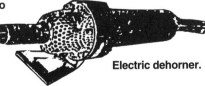

Electric dehorner.

Another method for dehorning young stock is to apply a caustic paste to the horn buds during the first 10 days of age. Although effective, the paste can sometimes get in the calf's eye in rainy weather, or may it may be rubbed or licked off by another animal. For these reasons, the paste treatment is not used very much unless the calf is isolated from other animals and in a protected area.

For animals under a year of age, a tube dehorner can be used to "scoop" the horn tissue away. In using this method, the dehorner is placed over the horn and twisted several times to cut into the base of the horn, then with a scooping motion, the horn is removed. Some bleeding will be present with this technique, but it can usually be controlled with a homeostatic powder or by pressure on the area with a cotton pad.

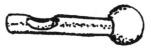

A tube dehorner.

Other instruments used for older animals are the Barnes dehorner, the Keystone dehorner, and the Dehorning saw. When dehorning older cattle, it is necessary to remove at least one fourth inch (six cm) of skin past the horn to prevent regrowth. Bleeding is to be expected with all of these methods. It can be controlled by cauterizing the vessels with a hot iron or by simply twisting or pulling the bleeding vessels with a forceps. To avoid problems with screwworms, it is very important to treat the area for several days with an effective repellent.

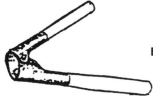

Barnes dehorner for older cattle.

Dehorning saw (used *only* for dehorning.)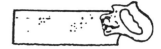

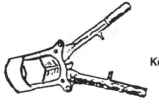

Keystone dehorner for older cattle.

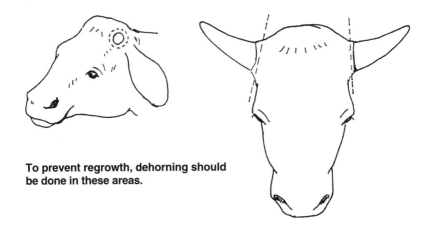

To prevent regrowth, dehorning should be done in these areas.

IDENTIFICATION

Identifying animals is done to keep track of individuals for records, proof of ownership, and quarantining sick animals. Several different methods can be used to accomplish this:

1. Branding is usually done with a hot iron. Proper restraint is very important when marking animals with this method. A special iron is heated red hot and pressed on the hide for at least three seconds. It is important that the animal be dry before applying the iron. When holding it on longer, there is a danger of creating a wound which could result in screwworm infection. An insect repellent should be applied if a wound results.

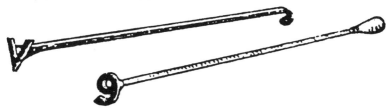

Branding Iron.

Another method of branding called "freeze branding" uses an iron which is super cooled using liquid nitrogen or some other gas. The resulting scar leaves a white mark where the iron was touched to the hide.

2. Ear tagging is an easy and quick method to perform. Either plastic or metal tags are placed in the ear with a special instrument with each tag having different numbers. A disadvantage of ear tags is they are often lost by coming loose or being torn from the ear.

3. Ear clipping is done by notching the ears using a preset pattern for identification.
4. Neck chains with an attached tag are an easy way to keep track of herd animals. Like ear tags, they are often lost over a period of time.
5. Tattooing the ears is used as a common method to identify those animals which have been vaccinated. It is done with an instrument that can be fitted with letters or numbers which are punched into the inside of the ear. Tattoo ink is then rubbed into the marks made by the instrument.

CULLING ANIMALS

As animals become older, they are less productive and consideration should be given to remove them from the herd. The age of cattle can be estimated from observing their front teeth.

The appearance or eruption of the permanent incisors or front teeth are as follows:

1. First pair..........................1 1/2 to 2 years.
2. Second pair.....................2 to 2 1/2 years.
3. Third pair.........................3 to 3 1/2 years.
4. Fourth pair.......................4 to 5 years.

THE ERUPTION OF TEETH IN CATTLE

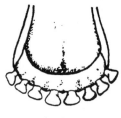
under 2 years

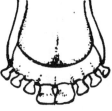
2 years 3 months

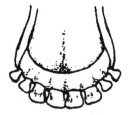
3 years

The small teeth are the temporary or milk teeth which fall out. The large teeth are permanent teeth.

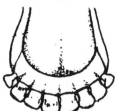
3 years 6 months

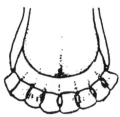
about 4 years old (4 pairs of permanent teeth)

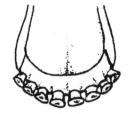
Old animal. 4 pairs of permanent teeth in wear.

Eruption of teeth.

As the animal ages past five years, the gums start to recede from the roots of the teeth. Using this method the age can be further estimated up to ten years of age according to the following:

1. First pair......................5 to 6 1/2 years.
2. Second pair..................6 1/2 to 7 1/2 years.
3. Third pair......................7 1/2 to 8 1/2 years.
4. Fourth pair....................8 1/2 to 10 years.

When using the teeth as a measurement of age, it is important to remember that variation exists between breeds and is influenced to some extent by the grazing conditions.

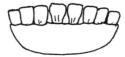 5-6 1/2 years

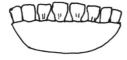 6 1/2-7 1/2 years

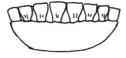 7 1/2-8 1/2 years

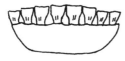 8 1/2-10 years

Most of the major management practices have been discussed above. There will be variations of these in each location according to custom and practice. When considering to raise either dairy or beef cattle, one should be aware of local conditions, facilities for handling, housing, labor available, feed sources, and disease problems.

Section X

Milking Management

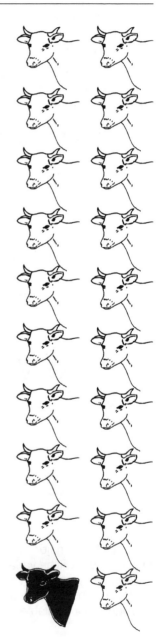

MILKING MANAGEMENT

The goal of milking management is to take milk from the udder of the cow in the most efficient and least damaging way. When electrical or mechanical power is available, milking machines can be used with great efficiency. In their absence, hand milking is the next choice. The average dairy cow is milked twice daily, although some dairyman may milk three times a day.

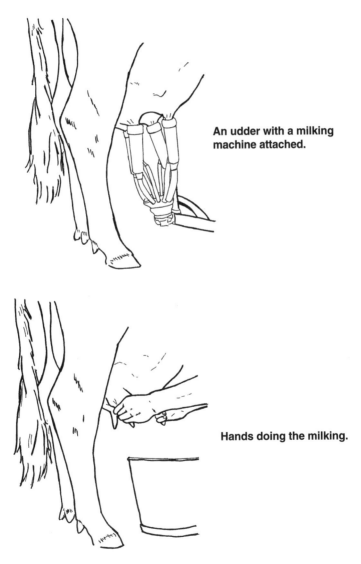

An udder with a milking machine attached.

Hands doing the milking.

To obtain the greatest milk production, calves should not be allowed to suckle the cows after the initial two to three days of obtaining colostrum. They can be hand fed milk from the cow or given a milk replacer using buckets or nipple bottles.

In preparing the cow for milking, it is important to wash the teats with a clean cloth and a mild antiseptic solution. A separate cloth should be used for each cow, then the teats should be dried before either hand or machine milking. The germs that cause mastitis (inflammation of the udder) can be easily transmitted from cow to cow if this procedure is not followed.

Hand milking of cows causes little damage to the teats. The milk is forced out by the pressure of the hands. Milking should be continued until the udder is slack and the teats no longer fill with milk. Milkers should wash, or at least rinse their hands between cows to prevent the spread of disease from cow to cow.

Milking machines have become popular in many parts of the world where the appropriate technology exists. While milking machines relieve the dairyman of much labor, there are many problems associated with their use. Very strict conditions must be used to assure the machines do not injure the teats and cause mastitis. As with any technology the pros and cons must be weighed to determine if installing machines to milk the cows will be a good investment. Perhaps the most important decision should revolve around:

1) Cost.
2) Available labor.
3) Technical support present.

Milking cows by machine, no matter the energy source, has requirements that make for efficient and non-harmful removal of milk. The literature on the requirements of milking machines is extensive and only an outline will be provided here.

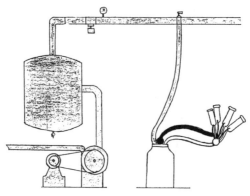

A milking machine.

The basics fundamentals of machine milking are related to a relationship between the following:

1) Vacuum (to draw the milk out).
2) Pulsations.
3) Massage pressure.

Vacuum is created in the system with a vacuum pump and the pressure at the teat end should be 10-12 inches of mercury equivalent. To maintain this level at the teat end, the vacuum pump needs to be able to move about 5 cubic feet per minute (CFM) for each milker unit.

Pulsation is necessary to massage the teat to force blood out of the teat tissues brought there by the vacuum pressure. The teat cup liner massages the teat when atmospheric air is allowed into the space between the liner and the shell. To properly stimulate blood flow out of the teat at least 8 inches of mercury pressure is necessary. The pulsator controls this admission of air. The number of times that this opening to atmospheric air occurs in one minute is the pulsator rate. The most common recommendation is about 60 pulsations per minute, but this can vary with each machine manufacturer.

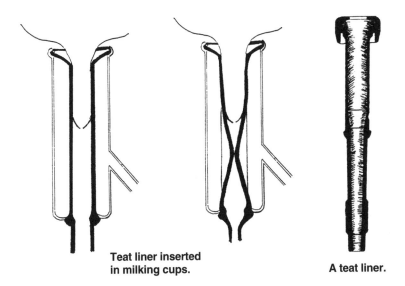

**Teat liner inserted
in milking cups.**

A teat liner.

The pulsation ratio is the time between the milking phase (liner is open and milk flows) and the massage, or resting phase (the liner is collapsed against teat and air is in the shell). This ratio varies with the manufacturer, but generally it is around 60 (milk):40 (rest).

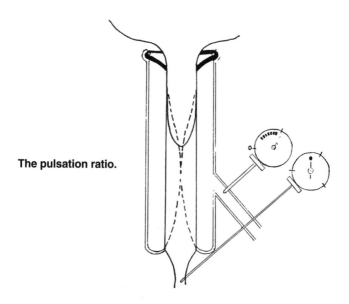

The pulsation ratio.

When there is inadequate massage and/or the milk rest ratio is too wide, the teat becomes swollen and damaged. This can lead to problems with milking and sometimes to mastitis. The vacuum level can also cause similar injury if it is at too high a level. It is regulated by a vacuum controller which is a weighted device in the vacuum supply line. Excessive vacuum can cause damage to the teat ends while inadequate vacuum will result in slow, incomplete milking with the teat cups possibly falling off.

To properly evaluate a milking machine system two important pieces of equipment are needed:

1) Air flow meter.

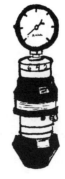

An air flow meter.

2) Vacuum recorder.

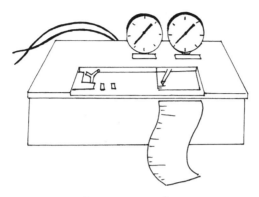

A vacuum recorder.

The airflow meter is an instrument to measure the cubic feet per minute capacity of a vacuum pump. The pulsator ratio and other functions in the milking system can be detected by using a vacuum recorder. A graphic recording is printed on paper to allow the operator to view the pulsator pattern and to judge the efficiency of the pulsators.

If the technology is available, milkings machines should be evaluated by the dairy farmer. There are many important factors to consider when making this very important decision. In addition to the cost of purchasing such equipment, it is very critical that a reliable support system be available for consultation and maintenance.

Section **XI**

Mastitis

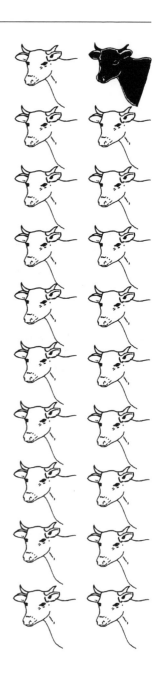

MASTITIS

In the dairy cow, mastitis is defined as an acute (rapid) or chronic (long lasting) inflammation of one or more mammary glands.

In dairyman's terms, mastitis is any inflammation of the udder. It occurs in two levels of severity: clinical and subclinical.

The clinical level is when changes in the milk occur such as flakes or clots, and the affected part of the udder is swollen, hot and sensitive. This form may be of short duration and be an individual cow problem. The animal may also go off feed and have an elevated temperature with the clinical signs of an illness.

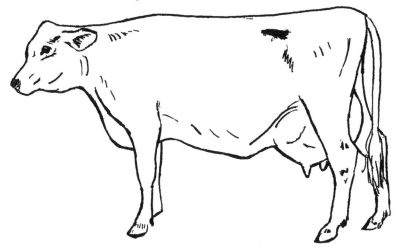

Cow with a swollen udder.

The subclinical or mild form of the disease may only cause slight changes in the milk, such as very small specks or flakes sometimes referred to as "garget". There may not be a noticeable change in the udder itself, although a reduction of milk in one or more quarters of the udder may occur. This form of the disease may clear up spontaneously without treatment. However, it may recur with swelling and heat in the udder in one or more quarters, and develop into the clinical form of mastitis.

In the treatment of mastitis, one of the first recommendations is to strip all the milk out of the affected quarters. This practice should be carried out frequently (every two or three hours) during the day. The animal should be made as comfortable as possible with dry, clean bedding. Warm packs may be applied to the affected part of the udder. Medication to reduce the temperature should be given. Supportive treatment to stimulate the appetite, such as vitamin injections, is helpful. These recommendations when carried out will do much to bring the infection under control.

In today's realm of veterinary treatments, there are medications available to inject into the infected udder through the teat canal. These are called udder infusions and should be used with special care and cleanliness. Follow directions on the label, and clean the teat with alcohol or another antiseptic before injecting the drugs.

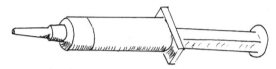

Udder infusion syringe.

Any infection in the glands of the udder will cause some damage to the gland tissue, and there will be a loss of the milk-secreting tissue. This loss may be very small and may not be detected by feel. At times the damage may be severe, resulting in the loss of one or more quarters. Regardless of the outcome of the damage, mastitis is a serious problem for the dairy industry.

As with all diseases, mastitis is best treated by prevention. This can start with the newborn calf. The teat ends of the new calf have a protective coating which prevents foreign materials from entering. This protection should remain in place until the animal delivers her first calf and the udder fills with milk. Therefore, an early prevention is to not allow young calves to suck each other's teats. This is a common practice when calves are housed together in groups. By separating the calves at birth and raising them in individual pens, this is eliminated.

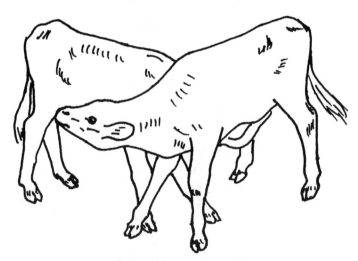

Calf sucking another calf.

It should be mentioned that when heifers have their first calf, and occasionally in heavy milking cows, there will be a swelling and inflammation which is called "mamitis". It should not confused with true mastitis as there is no bacterial invasion of the udder, but it can cause pain to the animal. This swelling can be reduced by frequent milking and massage. An ointment or balm applied to the udder also helps to reduce the swelling.

Udder edema, which is an accumulation of fluid associated with the udder, often occurs following calving. It is also not a disease like mastitis. Drugs and frequent milking are used to reduce the extra fluid from the body which is basically caused by a congestion of the blood flow associated with the udder.

The practice of good hygiene and careful attention to avoid damage to the teat ends are two very important practices to prevent mastitis. Another measure is to use a strip cup before milking to check for a visual presence of infection in the udder.

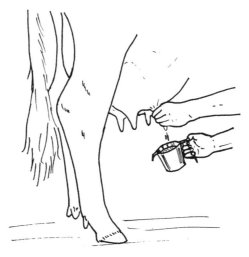

Strip cup being used.

Early detection and treatment can avoid costly chronic mastitis. Dipping the teats in an appropriate disinfectant after milking has also been shown to aid in the prevention of mastitis.

Section **XII**

Medical Care

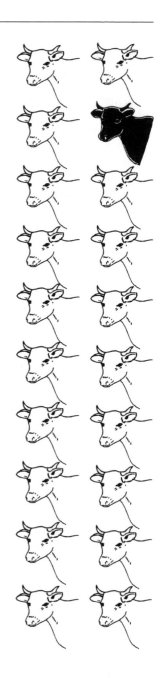

MEDICINE KIT FOR TREATING SICK AND INJURED ANIMALS

Every person who owns animals should have a medical kit to treat the most common problems that occur. Many of the illness and injuries of cattle can be handled by the farmer, or emergency first aid can be given while awaiting assistance.

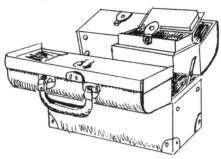

Medical bag

Some equipment necessary for examining and treating animals should include some or all of the following items:

For examination of the animal:
Strong rope and halter for restraint.
Nose tongs.
Flashlight.
Pencil and paper for important information.
Magnifying lens.

For wounds and infection of the skin:
Strong bandage rolls.
Cotton, sponges, or clean rags.
Soap and disinfectant for cleaning wounds.
Bucket or deep dish for water.
70% alcohol.
Hydrogen peroxide in a dark bottle.
White vinegar.
Iodine solution.
Petroleum jelly or vaseline in a jar or tube.
Antibiotic ointment.
Tick and fly repellent.
Scissors, knife, forceps, tweezers, surgical needles, and a suitable suture material.
Syringes and needles for injection.

For measuring the temperature:
Rectal thermometer.
For collecting samples:
Plastic bags or glass jars.
Plastic or glass tubes.
Scotch tape for collecting insects or worms.
For bacterial infections:
Penicillin for injection.
Tetracycline for injection.
Sulfa boluses for oral use.
Mastitis tubes for udder infusion.
For parasites:
Medicine for external and internal parasites. (See section on parasites for specific products)
For dehydration:
Prepackaged mix for rehydration.
Sodium bicarbonate, salt, and sugar for home mix.
Two examples of home mixes, if a commercial preparation is not available, are:
1. One litter of water mixed with two level tablespoons of honey or sugar, 1/4 teaspoon salt, and 1/4 teaspoon of baking soda (bicarbonate of soda).
2. Two liters of water mixed with one teaspoon of salt, one tablespoon baking soda, one can of beef consommé, and 1 pack of jam or jelly pectin.
For allergic reactions:
Epinephrine for injection.
Antihistamine for injection.
Corticosteroids for injection.

GENERAL WOUND TREATMENT

In any cattle operation owners will often be treating wounds from cuts, bites, horns, or other sharp objects. These injuries are often infected with bacteria and attract insects. A knowledge of wound treatment is essential when raising cattle.

One of the first concerns in treating an injury is to control bleeding if a clot has not already formed. The most common way is by direct pressure on the wound with a clean cloth or bandage. A rope or cord may also be tied above the cut to stop the blood circulation (this is a temporary measure). If the proper instruments are available, tweezers or forceps may be clamped on a vessel to stop the flow of blood or a small piece of string or fishing line can be used to tie around the "bleeder".

After stopping the bleeding, the wound should be washed with clean water and soap. The skin edges should be free of dirt and hair and the wound flushed several times with a mild disinfectant to remove all foreign material. A wound that is less than 12 hours old may be sutured. Wounds older than 12 hours should be left open to drain as bacteria have already contamined the area.

Daily treatments of open wounds with antibiotic powders along with a clean bandage, aid in the healing process. Salt applied directly to a wound is very irritating and should be avoided. However a saline solution of one teaspoon of salt in a cup of warm water is a simple but effective solution for cleaning wounds.

In tropical areas, screwworms infestation is a problem and should be avoided by placing a repellent around the edges of the wound to prevent flies from laying eggs.

Puncture wounds occur when a sharp object penetrates the skin and muscle. These are best treated by injections of antibiotics. Often the place where the skin was penetrated closes over and there is no drainage, resulting in an abscess or local infection.

To treat an abscess, the animal should be restrained, and the swelling probed with a large needle to see if pus is present. If so, the abscess can be opened with a sharp knife. The opening should be made at the lowest point of the swelling to allow adequate drainage. After the pus has been removed, a mild disinfectant should be flushed into the area for several days until healing has taken place. An antibiotic given by injection is helpful in treatment and a screwworm repellent should be placed around the opening. Deep puncture wounds are more likely to result in a more serious disease such as tetanus.

Broken bones should be dealt with on an individual basis. If the bone is broken in several places or protrudes through the skin, the chance for recovery is very poor. Such animals should be slaughtered for meat. Large animals (over 200 kg) with broken limbs rarely heal and should be considered for meat. In smaller animals or with a valuable animal, a decision may be made to treat the fracture. For a bone to heal, it must be brought into correct position and stabilized for at least six weeks. Various methods can be used to accomplish this, including splints, casts, and other supporting materials.

HOW TO USE MEDICINE

Drugs or medicines are substances that may be used in the treatment of diseases in animals. In many cases they may be necessary to save the life of an animal with a serious illness. When using these medications, it is important to remember that there can be harmful side effects to these drugs also, especially when not used properly. Allergic reactions can occur with certain drugs. Not all diseases will be affected by antibiotics, especially those caused by viruses. Antibiotics are most helpful in infections caused by bacteria.

Some general guidelines to use with drugs are:
Use the recommended drug for the specific disease problem.
Use drugs that are in date and that have been stored correctly.
Follow the recommendations on the label.
Give the correct dosage. Do not assume that increasing the dose may work better.
Be very clean when giving injections under the skin.
Boil syringes and needles in water for 15 minutes or soak then in a disinfectant solution before using.
Keep medicines cool and out of direct sunlight.

How to give medications:
Most common way is orally (by mouth).
Pill or bolus usually given with a balling gun.
Paste given with a syringe or paste gun.
Drench administered with a syringe, bottle, or stomach tube.
Orally mixed with feed or water.

The method used depends upon many things such as the disease being treated, the kind of drugs available, and the age of the animal.

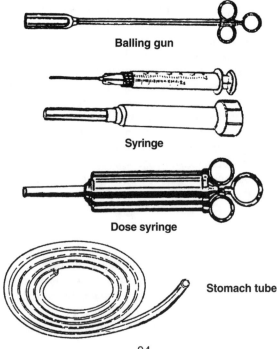

Balling gun

Syringe

Dose syringe

Stomach tube

Injection with a syringe and needle.

Subcutaneous injection is given under the skin, usually in the neck area. A short (1/2 to 1 inch- 1.25 to 2.55 cm) needle is best to use. The injection should be made at an angle.

Intramuscular injection is given in the muscle tissue. A longer needle, 1 1/2 inch (3.8 cm) is used. It is directed deep into the muscle usually in the neck, rump, or rear leg.

Intravenous injection is given into the vein. The jugular and tail vein are used most often. When using the jugular vein, the point of the needle should be directed against the flow of blood. Any medicine given in the blood must be given very slowly and the heart should be monitored closely. Care must be taken to give the medicine into the vein and not into the surrounding tissue.

Intra-peritoneal injection is placed directly into the abdominal cavity.

Most common injections:

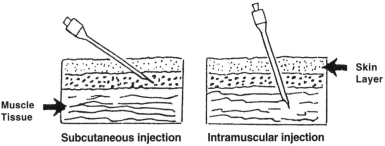

Muscle Tissue

Skin Layer

Subcutaneous injection   Intramuscular injection

When administrating injections, it is very important to follow the directions on the bottle. Caution should be taken to avoid accidental injection of oneself or another person. Some medicines should never be given in the blood stream, therefore when making an injection always pull back on the plunger of the syringe to check for the presence of blood before injecting. If blood appears, withdraw the syringe and use another site.

Some general guidelines to remember when using antibiotics are:

1. Antibiotics can be harmful as well as useful.
2. It is important to have an accurate diagnosis when giving antibiotics.
3. Remember that antibiotics are most effective against bacterial infections.
4. It is important to give the correct dosage at the recommended frequency and duration.
5. Withdrawal periods should be followed when treating animals that are producing milk or meat for human use.

6. To be most effective, antibiotics should be given early in the course of a disease.

A guide for telling if the antibiotic is working is to monitor the animals temperature. It should begin to return to normal within 24-48 hours after starting the medicine. If it does not, consider switching to another drug. Continue using the antibiotic for at least 48 hours after the temperature has returned to normal.

On occasion, an animal will have an allergic reaction to an antibiotic, or other drug. This is called "anaphylactic shock" and can result in death unless treated quickly. Agents most likely to cause this syndrome are penicillin products and vitamins, especially when injected into the blood stream.

The symptoms of shock are usually seen within a very short time after the drug has been given. They consist of nervous signs and restless behavior, followed by depression, vomiting, diarrhea, raised areas (wheals or hives) in the skin, salivation, and grinding of the teeth. Other findings are rapid, shallow breathing, sweating, convulsions, and muscle trembling.

Treatment of an animal in anaphylactic shock must be prompt. Injections of epinephrine, corticosteroids, and antihistamines are useful for reversing the signs and are usually life saving. Every medicine kit should contain anti-allergy medication since early treatment is so important.

CALCULATING DRUG DOSAGES

It is very important to have a basic understanding of how to calculate dosages of drugs when treating sick animals. If the correct amount of the drug is not given in a serious illness, the animal may not respond and die. Just as important as the correct dosage of a medication is the frequency and duration recommended by the manufacturer.

Drugs are measured in different methods according to how they are sold or manufactured. Some examples are:

1. Many medicines are weighed in grams (gms) and milligrams (mgs).

   Such as: 1000 milligrams (mg) equals 1 gram (gm) or 1 milligram (mg) which equals .001 gram (gm).

   An example of how a drug is measured is Tetracycline, which comes in a 500 mg capsule. It can also be written as:

   500 milligrams equals .5 gm.
   or 0.5 gm.
   or 0.500 gm.
   or 500 mg.

2. Many countries still weigh medicines in grains (grs). One grain equals 65 milligrams (mgs). One example is aspirin, which comes in a 5 grain tablet. Since each grain is the same as 65 mg, a 5 grain aspirin would equal 325 mg. (5 X 65 = 325).
3. Penicillin is often measured in units (u) or international units (IU). 1,600,000 units equal 1 gm or 1000 mg. Penicillin usually is sold in 400,000 units, which equal 240 mg.
4. Most liquids such as syrups, suspensions, and tonics are measured in milliliters or cubic centimeters. Examples of how they are used are:

One ml equals 1 milliliter (the same as one cc, which equals one cubic centimeter). Note that ml's and cc's are the same unit of measure.

1000 ml or 1000 cc equals 1 liter.

one teaspoon (tsp) equals five ml's or five cc's.

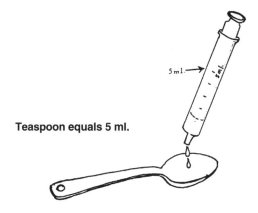

Teaspoon equals 5 ml.

Three teaspoons (tsps) equal one tablespoon (tbs), which equals 15 ml or 15 cc.

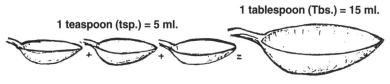

1 teaspoon (tsp.) = 5 ml.   **1 tablespoon (Tbs.) = 15 ml.**

3 teaspoons equals 1 tablespoon

Some teaspoons in the home may hold more or less than five ml's. When using a teaspoon for measuring medicine, it is important to know how much they hold. One way to determine what a spoon holds is to fill it with exactly five ml's of water using a syringe, and then make a mark

97

where the water comes to. Another way is to buy a spoon made to hold five ml's of liquid. Many medicines come with a spoon or holder that is marked for certain amounts which makes measuring easier.

If we want to give an animal the proper amount of drug we need to know three important facts:

1. The weight of the animal. This can be in kilograms (kg) or pounds (lb). Each kilogram equals 2.2 pounds. If the exact weight is not known, an estimate can be made with a heart girth measurement. In this method, a tape is placed around the chest of an animal at the point of the withers and heart. The tape is marked with numbers which give an estimate of the weight.

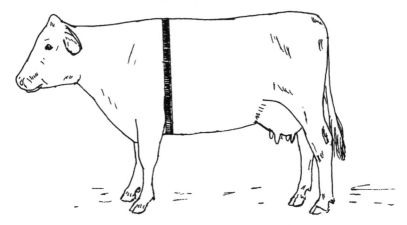

Measuring an animal to obtain the weight.

An estimate of an animal's weight can also be obtained by measuring the heart girth and using a table to determine the approximate weight. See Table 1.

Table 1. Estimated Live Weights of Cows from Heart Girths

Heart girth cm	Weight kg	Heart girth cm	Weight kg	Heart girth cm	Weight kg
140	255	160	328	180	409
142	264	162	338	183	420
145	273	165	348	185	431
147	282	168	358	188	442
150	291	170	368	190	453
152	300	173	378	193	464
155	309	175	388		
157	319	178	399		

2. Concentration of the drug. This can be found either on the bottle or in the package insert.
3. Dosage of the drug per kg or lb of body weight (BW). This can also be found on the package label or insert. It is usually expressed as mg/lb or mg/kg.

Once we know the above facts, we can calculate the correct dosage to administer to an animal. An example would be:

A farmer wishes to give tetracycline to a young calf for a lung infection. Using the above guidelines we would do the following:

1. Write down the weight of the animal. Assume the weight to be 45.5 kg or 100 lb.
2. If the dose is 5 mg/lb or 11 mg/kg, we would multiply the dose times the weight.

   (5 mg. X 100 lb. equals 500 mg. Or 11mg X 45.5 kg equals 500 mg.)
3. We would then need to figure how many ml's or cc's to give the animal. If there are 100 mg. in each ml or cc, we would divide the total mg's needed by the amount per ml.

********Total needed is 500 mg********
********Concentration is 100 mg. per ml********

Therefore: 500 divided by 100 equals five which in this case would be five ml's or cc's.

Using the above calculations, we would give the calf five ml's of tetracycline as a treatment for the lung infection.

It is very important to understand the method for calculating the proper amount of medicine to give to an animal. To gain confidence, one should practice using different examples. Having someone check the calculations is a good idea for the first few times until a high degree of confidence is reached.

Using the information listed in this section can prepare livestock owners to treat most of the common problems, which can occur. These basic skills are important in the overall program of keeping a healthy and productive herd and can be the difference between success and failure.

Section XIII

Diseases

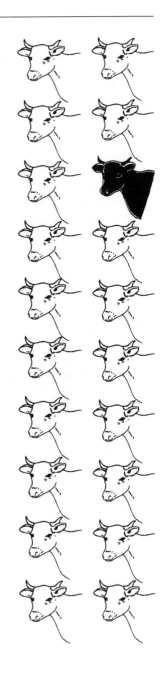

DISEASES

If an animal has a change from the normal function of the body, a disease or illness may be present. The major causes of disease are bacteria, viruses, protozoa, parasites, fungi, poisons, trauma, and poor nutrition.

Some of these agents are living organisms which can live outside or inside of an animal. They are spread by biting insects, direct contact between sick animals, and blood or secretions from infected animals.

Bacteria are very small one-celled organisms. They can live either inside or outside of an animal. Under certain conditions, bacteria can turn into very resistant spores which live for many years. Anthrax is an example of a spore forming bacteria. Mastitis, blackleg, navel ill, and calf diptheria are other examples of bacterial infections.

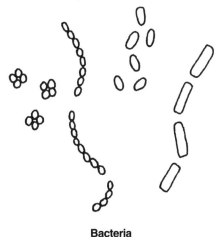

Bacteria

Viruses are smaller that bacteria. They can only be seen using very strong microscopes. They can only multiply inside an animal's body. Once they have entered a cell, to grow and multiply. Viruses tend to infect specific places in an animal's body. Rinderpest, African swine fever, and foot and mouth disease are examples of viruses.

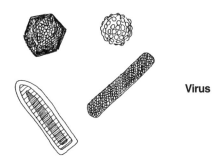

Virus

Protozoa are larger than bacteria and often use a tick or fly (intermediate host) to complete their life cycle. Some examples of diseases caused by protozoa are East Coast Fever and Redwater Tick Fever. Two examples of diseases that do not require an intermediate host to multiply are coccidiosis and trypanosomiasis.

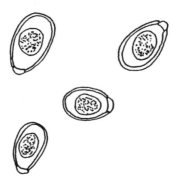

Protozoa

Another agent that causes disease is a rickettsia. It multiplies only in living cells. It is larger in size than bacteria. Anaplasmosis and heartwater are two examples of rickettsia.

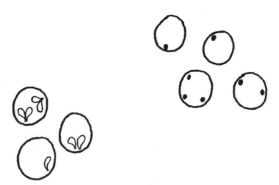

Rickettsia in Red Blood Cells

Parasites can often be seen with the eyes. They feed on another animal's blood or skin. Some of these live on the outside of the body and are called ectoparasites. Examples are ticks, mites, fleas, and lice. Others live in the body and are called endoparsites. These are blood flukes, flatworms, and roundworms.

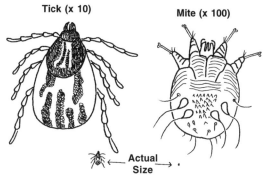

Tick (x 10)   Mite (x 100)

←— Actual Size —→ .

Ectoparasites (ticks, mites)

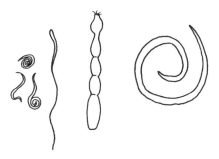

Endoparasites (flatworms, roundworms)

Fungi are members of the plant kingdom that can cause disease in animals. Ringworm is a common example. Fungi usually occur on the outside of the body.

Fungi (250-400x)

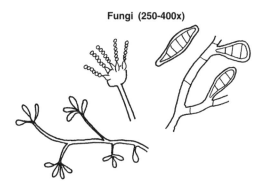

Fungi

HOW TO EXAMINE A SICK ANIMAL

To determine the cause of a sickness in an animal, begin by talking to the owner to determine the history. Find out how many animals are involved and what ages they are. Has there been an exposure to other animals recently? If so, what was the time period before the animals became sick? What are the signs of the illness, and how long does it last? Have any animals died? In general, the more information you can gather, the quicker a diagnosis can be made.

You should also observe the surroundings of the animals. Is the area clean and dry, or is it wet and marshy? Examine what the animals are eating. Some diseases are caused by poor quality feed or harmful plants.

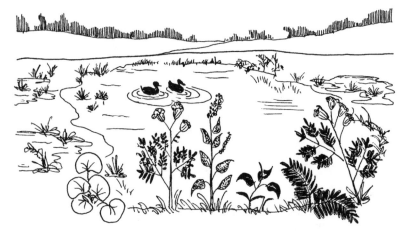

Wet marshy area and harmful weeds.

After asking questions, look at the sick animal very carefully. First, examine it from a distance noting the posture, alertness, and attitude. Note signs of difficult breathing, coughing, lameness, swelling, diarrhea or straining. An animal that does not want to get up or will not eat or drink may indicate a more serious problem.

Taking the temperature of an animal is an important part of the examination. To find the temperature, a thermometer must be used. Before using the thermometer, clean it with soap and water or alcohol. Shake it hard with a quick snap of the wrist until the silver line reads less than 36 degrees Centigrade or Celsius (C) or 98 degrees Fahrenheit (F). It is put in the rectum of the animal and left from one to three minutes before reading. The thermometer is read at the point where the silver line stops.

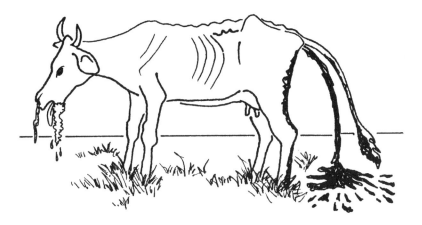

Sick cow.

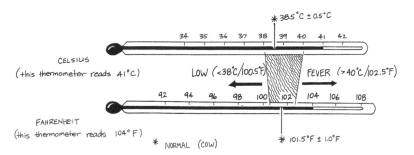

How to read the thermometer.

The normal temperature of cattle will vary from 38 degrees C to 38.5 degrees C or 101 degrees F to 102.5 degrees F. In younger animals this may increase by one degree. In most cases, an increase in body temperature usually indicates a disease. After using the thermometer, clean and store it in a protective case.

Observing the breathing (respiration) of an animal is another important part of the examination. In a healthy animal, the number of breaths per minute should be around 15-20. Pay attention to the way the animal breathes. Rapid shallow breathing can indicate pneumonia. Deep labored breathing is not normal. Observe if both sides of the chest move at the same time or if the breathing sounds are different on one side of the body.

To further examine the animal, you should note the haircoat, eyes, nose, and mouth for abnormal appearance. Any swellings should be noted. The digestive system can be evaluated by observing the movements of the paunch or rumen. This can be done by pushing a closed fist into the left upper flank region and holding a steady pressure in the area. Normal movements are from two to three per minute with alternating strong and weak contractions.

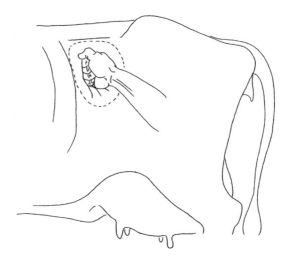

Person testing for rumen movements.

After a careful examination, a specific diagnosis should be made if possible. Sometimes it will be necessary to submit samples to a laboratory for analysis. Since some animal diseases can be transmitted to people, it is wise to take safety measures when collecting the samples.

DISEASE PREVENTION

Some diseases can be prevented in animals by the process of infecting the animal with a weak form of the causative agent. The term we use for this process vaccination. When an animal is vaccinated, special cells called antibodies are produced in the body. These cells attack disease agents that enter the body and can prevent disease from occurring.

Vaccines are not available for every disease, but when they are, it is a very easy way to prevent infection before it occurs.

In addition to using vaccines, the natural protection (immune system) an animal has can be made stronger by providing a clean environment, fresh, clean water, and a well balanced nutritional program. Strong, healthy animals can resist disease better than weak ones.

Section XIV

Bacterial Diseases

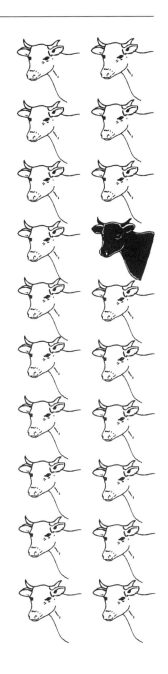

BACTERIAL DISEASES

ANTHRAX (Fievre Charbonneuse, Carbunco Bacteridiano)

Anthrax, caused by *Bacillus anthracis,* is found throughout the world and can infect all warm-blooded animals including man. It is seen more during the rainy season and in tropical areas.

Eating contaminated animal products or drinking water containing the anthrax bacteria is the usual means of infection. The organism can also enter the body through the respiratory tract or via an open wound. An important fact about anthrax is that the bacteria can form spores which are very resistant and can remain infective for 10-20 years in the environment.

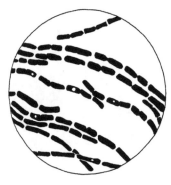 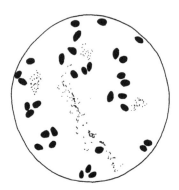

Anthrax organism   Anthrax spore

Often the only sign of anthrax in cattle is sudden death without any warning signs. When symptoms are noticed they include; high fever, difficult breathing, stumbling, trembling, and convulsions. Bloody discharge is often seen from the nose and rectum. Other conditions which may cause sudden death, like anthrax, are snake bite, lightning strike, or bloat.

An animal suspected of dying from anthrax should have an accurate diagnosis with the help of laboratory techniques. To avoid contamination of the area, it is best not to perform an autopsy. A blood smear from the ear or tail will serve as a diagnostic aid. The blood from an animal dying from anthrax is very dark and not clotted.

It is very important not to eat meat from an animal that may have died from Anthrax, as this could result in human deaths. Vaccines are available for use in areas where anthrax is present.

Treatment is rarely successful, but penicillin is the drug most often used. Animals dying of anthrax should be either burned or buried on the spot and a disinfectant such as quick lime applied to the area.

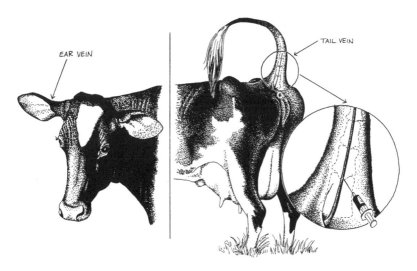

Taking a blood smear from the tail or ear.

CLOSTRIDIAL DISEASES *(Gas forming diseases)*

There are several different diseases in cattle caused by bacteria from this group. The damage to animals from this organism results from the production of toxins within the tissue which are very harmful. Most types of clostridial bacteria produce spores which like anthrax can remain infective for many years.

BLACKLEG *(Black Quarter, Quarter III, Charbon Symptomatique, Felon, Carbunco Symtomatico)*

This disease is caused by a bacterium called *Clostridium chauvoei (feseri)*. It is usually seen in younger animals from 6-24 months of age. The organism is found naturally in the intestinal tract but does not normally cause disease. Infection results when the spores gain entrance into the body through an injury or by being ingested. Once inside the body in spore form the bacteria enter the blood stream and begin to multiply in muscle tissues. The toxin produced by the bacteria results in a severe reaction especially to the heavy muscled areas of the body. If symptoms are observed before death, they include swellings on the upper legs, which crackle when touched due to gas under the skin, and lameness. Affected animals are very depressed, have a high fever, and may have bloody discharges from the nose and rectum before and after death. Treatment is usually not successful, however large doses of penicillin may be of value in early cases.

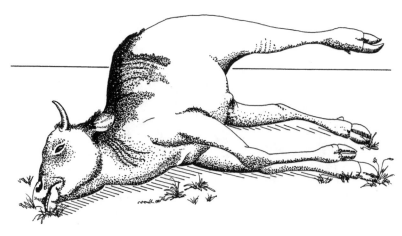

Animal with swollen leg muscle.

Because blackleg resembles anthrax, it is important to obtain an accurate diagnosis with a blood smear using laboratory techniques. An autopsy should not be done. Disposal of the body should be made using the same precautions as with anthrax because of the risk of contamination of the soil.

A very effective vaccine is available and should be used in all areas where this disease occurs, especially in young animals.

MALIGNANT EDEMA (Gangrenous Septicemia)

This disease is caused by *Clostridium septicum*. It is closely related to blackleg. It most often occurs following a wound such as castration where the bacteria gain entrance to the tissue. Like blackleg, it is a very serious infection and almost always causes death which may be preceded by high fever, depression, and swelling of the affected muscle tissue.

Treatment is similar to that of blackleg as well as the method of diagnosis. The carcass should be burned or buried to avoid contamination of the soil. An effective vaccine is available.

ACUTE CERVICAL HEMORRHAGIC EDEMA

Clostridium sordelli is the cause of this disease and is very similar to malignant edema except there is usually not a wound present for the bacteria to enter the body. The signs are similar to the other clostridial infections such as high fever, depression, loss of coordination, and rapid death. The most common lesions found are swellings and dark pockets of blood in the neck area. Penicillin is the drug of choice for treatment but is rarely successful. For prevention, a vaccine is available.

TETANUS *(Lockjaw, Tatanos)*

The bacteria *Clostridium tetani* is the cause of tetanus. It is almost always fatal to domestic animals and man. The organism usually enters the body through deep wounds or surgical procedures such as castration. Early signs of the disease include muscle stiffness and spasms of the body. The jaw muscles are very tense and hold the mouth together (lockjaw), and the tail and ears will usually be stiff. With the jaw muscles being affected, the animal cannot eat or drink. They are also very sensitive to light and sound and are often are observed in a saw-horse position.

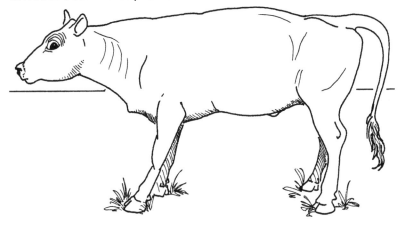

Saw-horse stance of an animal, raised tail, and ears.

With early treatment, some animals can be saved. An injection of tetanus antitoxin is helpful as well as cleaning and disinfecting of the wound. Large doses of penicillin are necessary treatment of tetanus. It is important to be very clean when performing surgical procedures such as castration and dehorning, as a preventive measure. A vaccine is available for animals as well as humans.

BOTULISM *(Lamziekte Disease)*

Botulism, which is a fatal disease affecting the nervous system, is caused by *Clostridium botulinum*. It is caused by eating contaminated feed or water in Which the organism is found. Early signs include staggering, swallowing difficulties, drooling, vacant stare, and a generalized paralysis including the mouth and tongue. A weakness of the muscles of respiration usually results in death within one to four days. Treatment is not very effective. Prevention includes a proper diet (avoiding spoiled or poorly prepared food), fresh water, and general cleanliness. A vaccine is available for use in problem areas.

ENTEROTOXEMIA (Overeating Disease)

Enterotoxemia is seen in two forms, that of nursing calves fed supplemental grain and in cattle on lush feed and concentrates. It is caused by an organism called *Clostridium perfrigens* type C & D. In young nursing calves the symptoms develop rapidly, resulting in death in a few hours. If signs are noted, they include bloat, abdominal pain, diarrhea, depression, and fever. The cause is often overeating, which results in indigestion, allowing the bacteria to grow in large numbers in the intestines. A toxin is released when the organisms begin to die which causes the damage to the body. Treatment consists of clostridium antiserum, antihistamines, and penicillin. A vaccine is available.

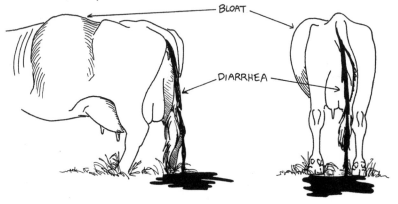

Animal with bloat and diarrhea.

The other form of the disease is with animals on high energy food. The signs usually appear within a short time after eating a large amount of grain. Signs and treatment of the illness are similar to those found with nursing calves. Prevention is the best measure. Reducing the exposure to high energy feeds, and regular feeding times are helpful.

BLACK DISEASE (Infectious Necrotic Hepatitis)

Clostridium novyi type B is the cause of this clostridial disease which affects the liver resulting in a high death rate. Signs include fever, depression, and death in a short time. Liver flukes are often found on necropsy and may contribute to the course of the disease. Antibiotics can be used as a treatment but are usually not very effective. Vaccines are available for prevention.

BACILLARY HEMOGLOBINURIA

This is a disease that is usually fatal and has signs similar to black disease. It is caused by *Clostridium haemolyticum*. Often the urine has a reddish color and the membranes may be yellow indicating liver damage. Treatment and control measures are the same as for black disease. Vaccines should be used as a preventive measure.

DISEASES AFFECTING THE RESPIRATORY TRACT

TUBERCULOSIS (Pearl's Disease, Phthisis, Consumption)

This disease is found in all parts of the world but is more common in tropical regions of Africa and South America. It affects almost all species of animals as well as man. There are three distinct types of tuberculosis. They are human, bovine and avian, and all are caused by bacteria in the genus *Mycobacterium*. Cross infection can occur in some animals from one species to another.

Transmission from sick to healthy animals is mainly by breathing or ingesting infected material. Sick animals often have a cough or diarrhea, which spreads the bacteria in the environment.

Signs of an animal with tuberculosis will vary according to where the bacteria are growing in the body. With a slow loss of weight, a chronic cough, and enlargement of lymph nodes, the disease should be suspected. Milk production will be less than normal and hard swellings may be felt in the udder. Diarrhea is usually present if the organism is affecting the intestines.

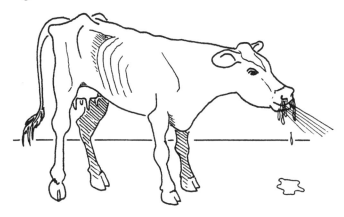

Skinny cow with a cough.

Since most affected animals die from the disease, a diagnosis is often made from an autopsy. There are usually hard pus filled lumps found wherever the bacteria were growing. The lungs are involved most often, although any organ in the body may be infected. While the animal is alive, a skin test can be used for identifying infected animals. This test is very useful in the control of tuberculosis as reactors to the

113

"tuberculin" test can be removed from the herd, reducing the spread of the disease. Treatment is not recommended due to the contagious nature of the disease. Since humans are susceptible to tuberculosis, care should be taken when handling infected meat, milk, or tissues. Milk intended for human consumption should be boiled (pasteurized).

CONTAGIOUS BOVINE PLEUROPNEUMONIA *(Peri-Pneunmonia)*

This is a highly infectious disease which causes a severe infection of the lungs. It is caused by an organism called *Mycoplasma mycoides*. Its occurrence is widespread in certain regions of Africa, Australia, Asia, and Latin America. Mainly cattle and buffalo are affected. The incubation period ranges from one to four weeks. Infected animals show signs related to pneumonia and pleurisy (the membrane lining of the chest cavity). Fever, coughing, and labored breathing are common symptoms along with depression, reduced appetite, and a swelling in the neck and throat. The disease often has a long duration with the animal showing bouts of diarrhea, then constipation. In the latter stages, breathing becomes very difficult and painful. The course of the infection ranges from 1-7 weeks with some animals recovering but remaining chronic shedders of the organism.

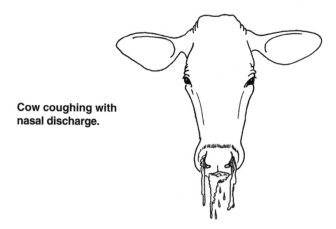

Cow coughing with nasal discharge.

Diagnosis of the disease is based on the typical signs, postmortem and laboratory findings. Treatment is not recommended, due to the animals possibly harboring live organisms in the lungs and spreading the infection to other animals. Control is based on diagnosis, quarantine, slaughter, and vaccination.

DIPHTHERIA *(Bacillary Necrosis)*

This is a disease affecting mostly young calves caused by the bacterium *Fusiformis necrophorus*. It is found throughout the world. Symptoms can start as early as three days of age in calves and will include coughing, salivation, high fever, and the occurrence of a slimy yellowish deposit in the mouth. A foul smell develops from the sticky, rope-like membranes which are firmly attached to the tissues. Often the face will appear swollen and ulcers may be found on the tongue. Even though the animals breathe with a loud snoring sound, they are usually not depressed.

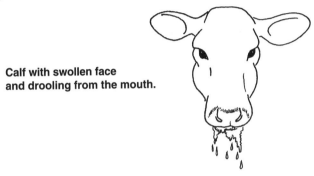

**Calf with swollen face
and drooling from the mouth.**

Diagnosis is made by observing the typical signs and from examination of the mouth. Some cases may lead to pneumonia but this is not very common, especially if antibiotics are used in the early stages. Coarse feed should be avoided during the active course of the disease.

FOOT ROT *(Foul in the Foot, Panartium, Pietin)*

This infection of the feet of animals, which is world wide in occurrence, is caused be an organism called *Fusiformis necrophorus*. Living in the soil, the bacteria gains entrance through the skin from an injury. It is occurs most often in damp, wet conditions.

The first symptoms noted are lameness of usually one foot. Swelling develops above the hoof, and the area between the claws becomes red and tender as the disease progresses. An abscess may result from the infection. In long standing cases, the tendons and joint may become involved resulting in permanent lameness.

Treatment is usually successful if started early in the infection by using antibiotics, cleaning the affected area, and disinfecting the tissue. A foot bath can be used in which affected animals walk through a solution such as 2-5% copper sulfate, 4% formaldehyde, or a powder

**Cow with a swollen foot.
Also an enlarged view of
the infected foot and joint.**

of copper sulfate and slaked lime. It is important to provide a dry area for the animals as a control measure.

HEMORRHAGIC SEPTICEMIA
(Pasteurellosis, Shipping-Fever, Cattle Fever)

This disease, which occurs mainly in cattle in stress related conditions, is caused by a combination of factors. It is thought that a viral infection weakens the animal which lowers the body's resistance. Pasteurella organisms normally found in the nasal passages multiply in large numbers causing the symptoms seen in hemorrhagic septicemia.

Since this is a disease of world wide distribution, it is difficult to control. It affects all domestic ruminants as well as those in the wild. Buffalo are very susceptible to this disease.

The symptoms of hemorrhagic septicemia are mostly related to the respiratory system. There is a persistent cough and swelling occurs in the throat and chest area. Diarrhea may also occur as well as a high fever. Some cases recover quickly while others are long lasting infection.

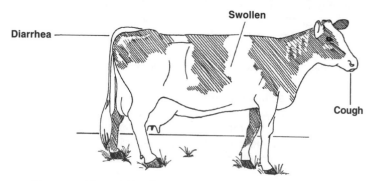

Cow coughing and having diarrhea. Chest and throat are swollen.

Diagnosis of the disease is made on the basis of the severe respiratory symptoms. Post-mortem findings include bloody areas under the skin, on the intestines and heart. A sticky yellow fluid is often lining the chest and abdominal cavities, and in the muscle tissues. A history of stressful conditions just before the illness began may be helpful in identifying the disease.

If caught in the early stages, treatment with antibiotics is usually effective. Since it is so important to begin treatment quickly, it is a good idea to monitor the temperature of any animal suspected of getting the disease. A vaccine is available which reduces the infection level. Care should be taken to eliminate conditions of stress such as overcrowding, poor nutrition, and exposure to bad weather.

DISEASES AFFECTING REPRODUCTION

BRUCELLOSIS (Contagious Abortion, Bang's Disease, Undulant Fever, Epizootic Abortion, Malta Fever)

One of the features of brucellosis is the large number of abortions it can cause in a herd of cattle. The causative organism, *Brucellosis abortus* affects the reproductive tract of mainly cattle and buffaloes, although all animals as well as man are susceptible. Once infected, an animal can shed the bacteria via the uterus, fetus, fetal membranes, testicles, and through the milk for up to two years. It occurs throughout the world.

In humans the infection is called undulant fever. It is most often transmitted by drinking affected milk or from exposure to the organisms from infected aborted tissue or associated discharges. Symptoms in man include a fever which comes and goes, along with sweating and general weakness. A diagnosis can be made from a laboratory test of the blood.

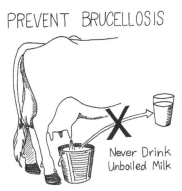

PREVENT BRUCELLOSIS

Never Drink
Unboiled Milk

Cow with milk bucket under the udder. "Prevent brucellosis, never drink unboiled milk."

117

To prevent brucellosis, strict guidelines should be followed. The most important are:

1) Test all new animals entering the herd.
2) Discard all infected tissue by burning or burying.
3) Boiling milk before drinking (pasteurizing).
4) Using latex or plastic gloves when assisting in calving.
5) Notifying government authorities if brucellosis is suspected.

VIBRIOSIS (Bovine Genital Campylabacteriosis)

Vibrosis in a disease which is found primarily in the reproductive tracts of both male and female cattle. It is caused by an organism called *Campylobacter* (Vibrio) fetus and occurs world wide.

This infection is spread mainly by breeding with infected bulls. The symptoms are low pregnancy rates and reduced fertility. Any time there are a large number of cows coming back in heat after breeding, vibriosis should be suspected. Abortions are rare.

Laboratory tests are available for diagnosis in the individual animal, but a careful history is the usual method of locating the problem.

Treatment of individual cows is usually not done. The best control is by using artificial insemination of semen from clean bulls and a period of sexual rest for the cows. If natural breeding is used, bulls should be tested and treated before exposure to the herd. A vaccine is available if preventative measures are not effective.

LEPTOSPIROSIS (Redwater of Calves)

All species of animals, including man, can be infected with this bacteria of the *Leptospira species*. It is found throughout the world and is spread most often by contact with infected urine. Drinking water is an important source of transmission with rodents often being a source of the disease.

The signs of leptospirosis are usually more severe in young animals. In calves, the urine may be bloody and the mucous membranes may be yellow due to liver damage. Older cattle may have bloody milk and abortions late in pregnancy. Diagnosis is usually made on the basis of blood and urine tests of infected animals with a history of abortions and bloody mastitis in older cattle.

Since the most common source of infection is from drinking water, care should be taken to provide clean water and effective rodent control. Infected swine are also responsible for transmitting leptospirosis to cattle. A strict separation of these two species should be made if possible.

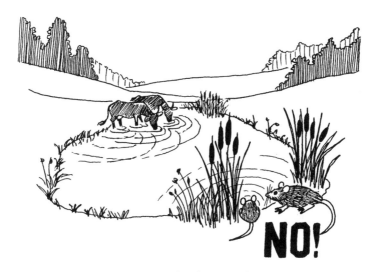

Rat drinking from pond.

Additional measures for control include disposing of infected material by burning or burial. Affected milk should also be discarded and not used for feeding calves or human consumption.

A vaccine is available and should be used in areas where leptospirosis is present.

ACTINOMYCOSIS *(Lumpy Jaw)*

This is a disease that affects a wide variety of domestic animals as well as man. It is caused by a bacteria called *Actinomyces bovis* which is found normally in the mouth and skin. Infection is thought to occur through wounds. Affected areas are most often found in the bony areas of the jaw and head.

The main sign is swelling on the upper and lower jaw with draining tracts of pus coming through the skin. Scar tissue may be present and eating may be difficult due to loose infected teeth.

Treatment involves surgery when the infection is localized, followed by flushing with iodine solution or streptomycin. Once the bony areas become affected, treatment is very difficult. Injections of streptomycin or sulfa drugs will slow the advancement of the disease but a cure is unlikely.

ACTINOBACILLOSIS *(Wooden Tongue)*

This is a similar disease to lumpy jaw but is found primarily in soft tissues, especially the tongue in cattle. The organism causing the symptoms is *Actinobacillus lignieresi*.

119

Affected animals experience difficulty in eating and chewing due to the swollen and inflamed tongue. At times it will protrude from the mouth and interfere with drinking. Treatment is usually successful, and often dramatic. Injections of intravenous sodium iodine, as well as other antibiotics such as streptomycin, and oxytetracyclines can be used.

PINKEYE (Infectious Bovine Keratoconjunctivitis)

This is an infection of one or both eyes that is caused by a bacteria called *Moraxella bovis*. It is spread by direct contact from an infected animal or by insects. It is world wide in occurrence.

When an animal is first infected, there is a watery discharge from the eyes. As the disease progresses, the eye may become cloudy and the eyelids may swell. In advanced cases, the eye may develop an ulcer and rupture, resulting in blindness.

In the diagnosis of pinkeye, it is important to note that only the eye is affected. Other diseases such as Infectious Bovine Rhinotrachities (IBR), Bovine Virus Diarrhea (BVD), and Malignant Catarrah Fever (MCF) involve other parts of the body as well as the eye.

Treatment for the organism should be started early to avoid damage to the eye. Antibiotics should be placed directly in the eye for best results. It is preferable to avoid direct sunlight and insects while the eye is infected.

Control of flies and ticks is an important part of preventing pinkeye. A vaccine is available to prevent serious outbreaks.

Section **XV**

Viral Diseases

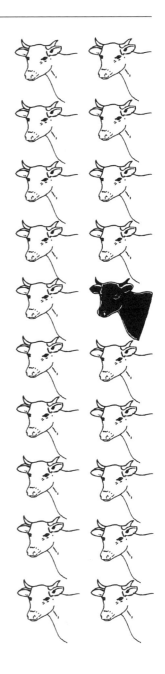

DISEASES CAUSED BY VIRUSES

FOOT AND MOUTH DISEASE (F.M.D., Afta Epizootica, Afthosa Fie-vre', Aphteuse)

This is a very contagious disease affecting mostly cattle and other split hoof (cloven hoof) animals. It is very common in the tropics, especially South America, Africa, and Asia. At this time North America, Australia, and New Zealand are free of the disease.

The most serious harm from foot and mouth disease is reduced production of affected animals. Its ability to spread rapidly to other animals is also of great concern.

The symptoms of the disease will generally appear in an animal within three to eight days after exposure to the virus. It can be spread by the milk, urine and nasal discharge by direct contact. Wild animals, including birds, can transmit the infectious agent from farm to farm. A high temperature and loss of appetite are an early sign of the infection which progresses to blisters or vesicles on the tongue and feet. Affected animals become lame and have difficulty swallowing. The teats and udder are also affected, resulting in loss of milk production. Young animals will often have heart damage, and either die or never grow normally. Within 7-14 days affected animals will generally recover.

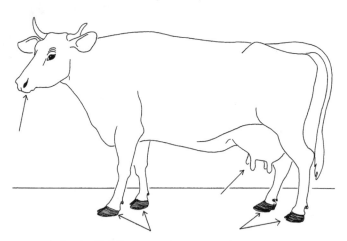

Animal with blisters on the tongue, feet, and teats.

It is important to make an accurate diagnosis of Foot and Mouth Disease because of its impact on the animal industry. Another disease called Vesicular Stomatitis resembles Foot and Mouth Disease very closely. Government authorities must be contacted to establish the true identity of the disease.

Treatment is usually limited to drugs to control the symptoms.
Vaccines are available but do not always give total protection due to the different sub-types of viruses which cause the disease. The only sure means of control is by slaughter of all affected animals.

VESICULAR STOMATITIS (V.S., Sore Mouth, Stomatite Vesiculeuse Contagiuse)

Vesicular stomatitis (V.S.) is similar to foot and mouth disease but it does not have the same economic importance. It affects horses, cattle, and swine. Almost all countries have V.S. present.

After exposure to the virus, symptoms appear in 3-5 days which include fever and blisters in the mouth and tongue. The teats and feet are not usually involved.

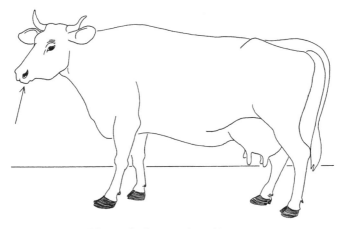

Blisters in the mouth and tongue.

Since it is difficult to tell the difference between V.S. and F.M.D. in the early stages, government officials should be notified when animals are found to show signs of either disease.

The recovery period from V.S. is generally rapid and there are very few side effects. Treatment is usually not indicated. A vaccine has been developed but is not in wide use.

MALIGNANT CATARRHAL FEVER (M.C.F., Malignant Head Catarrh, Snotsiekte)

Malignant Catarrhal Fever (M.C.F.) is a very serious disease which occurs world wide but it is more widespread in East, Central, and

123

South Africa. It is fatal to cattle, buffalo, and deer. Some wild ruminants as well as sheep and goats may not show signs of the disease, but are thought to be carriers of the virus.

After exposure to the infection, it may take up to four months for signs of the disease to appear. Symptoms associated with M.C.F. are mainly related to the respiratory tract, but diarrhea and blindness may also be present as well as nervous signs. Affected animals will usually die within a short time after being sick.

Very little can be done to treat the disease. Control is mainly by keeping healthy animals away from wild game as well as goats and sheep.

RINDERPEST (R.P.,Cattle Plague, Peste Bovina)

Once considered the world's most destructive disease of cattle, Rinderpest (R.P.) is now contained in East and West Africa, the near East, and Asia. It is highly contagious and usually deadly to all ruminants and swine.

After 3 to 15 days from initial exposure to the virus of R.P., the signs of the disease begin to appear. They include high fever, depression, and inflammation of the mouth and eyes. Ulcers appear in the mouth and a foul smelling breath is noted. There is usually a ropy, yellow discharge from the nose along with rapid breathing and coughing. Diarrhea usually follows the respiratory signs. Death is close to 100% of those affected.

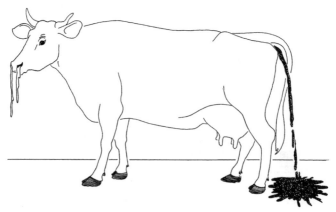

Ropy discharge from nose and diarrhea.

A laboratory diagnosis may be necessary to confirm the disease. Treatment is usually not helpful. A vaccine is available and is effective for life. In areas where R.P. is present, all susceptible animals should be vaccinated at six months of age. Because the disease affects wild animals which are difficult to vaccinate, the disease is very hard to control.

BOVINE VIRAL DIARRHEA (B.V.D.,Mucosal Disease)

Ruminants, both domestic and wild, throughout the world are susceptible to Bovine Viral Diarrhea (B.V.D.). Younger animals usually are affected more than adults. Although the infection rate can be high, very few animals die from the disease.

Sick animals show signs of fever, blisters and ulcers in the mouth along with diarrhea. Pregnant animals will often abort 3 to 6 months after infection or give birth to calves with nervous signs.

Since the symptoms of B.V.D. are similar to R.P. and F.M.D. it is important to have a laboratory diagnosis. Treatment is usually not successful. A vaccine is available.

COW POX (Variola)

This is a viral disease which affect the cells of the skin. It is primarily a disease of cattle, but can be transmitted to man, usually during the act of milking.

Cow Pox affects the thinner, hairless parts of the body of cattle such as the udder and teats. Blisters usually appear which break and become infected. Scabs then form and leave a scab or "poc" mark. The first signs appear 3 to 5 after exposure and usually will heal after 10 to 14 days.

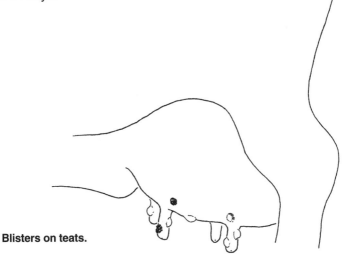

Blisters on teats.

Treatment involves cleaning the local sores and applying a protective ointment. A vaccine is available but is not used very often since the signs are very mild. Keeping the hands and milking equipment clean is the best control measure.

WARTS (Papillomas or Fibromas)

Warts appear primarily on young animals. They are fleshy growths which occur around the head, neck, udder, and prepuce. Most warts will go away without treatment as the animal matures. Vaccines are available from commercial sources or a vaccine can be made by using the warts from the affected animal. Warts that become large on an animal can be surgically removed.

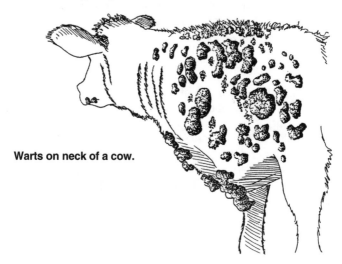

Warts on neck of a cow.

INFECTIOUS BOVINE RHINOTRACHEITIS
(I.B.R., Infectious Pustular Vulvovaginitis-I.P.V.)

This is a viral disease that is world wide in ruminants. It is unique in that the same virus can produce different signs in animals. Recovered animals usually remain carriers and continue to spread the disease by close contact or through reproduction.

The respiratory signs of I.B.R. usually appear within seven days after exposure. A high fever, runnny eyes, nasal discharge, and loss of appetite are common. Pregnant animals usually abort and unless there are complications, sick animals will recover in 10-14 days.

The reproductive form of the virus, I.P.V. consists of low fever and congestion and redness of the vagina and vulva. There may be a discharge and small blisters present in the vagina. Bulls often show an infection of the prepuce and penis. Most of the signs will disappear in 10-14 days. Look for sores in the vulva in the cow and the prepuce in the bull.

Because this disease may be mistaken for more serious economic sickness, it is important to obtain an accurate diagnosis by laboratory methods. A vaccine is available for prevention but it should not be given to pregnant animals as abortion may occur. Treatment is usually for secondary infections.

RABIES (Mad Cow, Hydrophobia, Lyssa, Rage)

Rabies is one of the most feared diseases of man and animals. It affects the nervous system and is almost always fatal. There is a world wide distribution of rabies except for the British Isles, Hawaii, Australia, and New Zealand. It is most often transmitted by the bite of an affected animal, most commonly dogs, cats, skunks, foxes, hyenas, mongoose, and bats.

From the time of exposure of the virus until signs of the disease appears it can be 3-8 weeks to six months or more. In cattle the early symptoms are often a change of behavior and increased in excitability. Their voice will change and they may bellow excessively. In the later stages, there will be grinding of the teeth and excess salivation. Weakness in the hindquarters and a generalized paralysis precede death.

Important signs include:
1. Change of behavior.
2. Excited and nervous.
3. Excessive bellowing.
4. Salivation.
5. Weakness and paralysis.
6. Death.

Because of the danger to humans, the proper health authorities should be notified if rabies is suspected in an animal. Once the symptoms of rabies have started, there is no treatment. If there has been a human exposure, it is important to start the preventative vaccine as soon as possible. A vaccine is available for animals and man to prevent rabies.

Section XVI

Protozoan Diseases

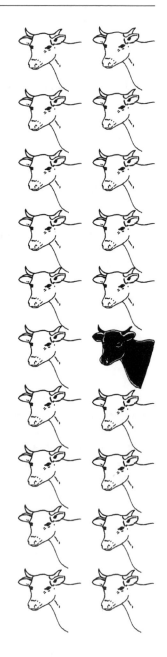

PROTOZOAN DISEASES

There are three major diseases affecting cattle that are caused by protozoal organisms. One is trypanosomiasis which is transmitted by the tsetse fly and other biting insects. The other two are trichomoniasis, an infertility disease, and coccidiosis which causes diarrhea, especially in young animals.

TRYPANOSOMIASIS (Nagana, Sannare, Sleeping Sickness, Chagas Disease)

Trypanosomiasis is the name given for a group of diseases caused by a protozoa from the genus *Trypanosoma (T. congolense, T. vivax)* In Africa the disease is spread by the tsetse fly. It also occurs in Central and South America where it is transmitted by other insect vectors such as biting flies.

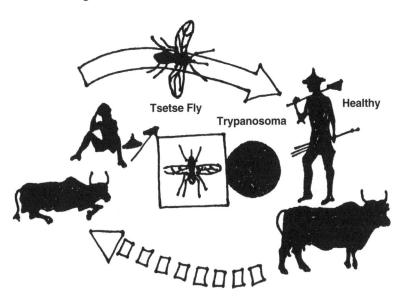

Cycle of African trypanosomiasis.

Central Africa is the area affected most by trypanosomiasis. Tsetse flies are present in an area of over 4.5 million square miles (approx. 9 million square kilometers) in the heart of rich agriculture land. The threat of disease is always present for millions of cattle and over 35 million people. Because of its economic importance, it is one of the most serious diseases found in Africa.

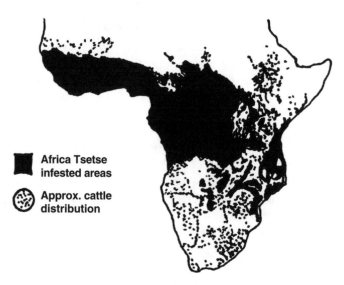

◼ Africa Tsetse
infested areas

🌐 Approx. cattle
distribution

Tsetse fly infested areas and cattle distribution.

The tsetse fly is a critical factor in the spread of nagana and sleeping sickness in Africa. It is in the fly that the infective stage of the protozoan develops. Since the female must have a blood meal before breeding, the infection is passed on to the next host by way of the salivary glands during feeding. In other countries, the disease is transferred through mechanical means, such as biting flies, carrying the infectious trypanosomes from one animal to another.

In nature the disease is spread mainly from animals such as the warthog and giraffe which have developed an immunity but remain carriers of the infectious organism. All species of domestic animals are susceptible to trypanosomiasis including man.

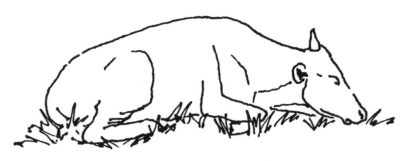

Cow with trypanosomiasis.

130

At the time of infection until symptoms appear is only five to seven days. The early signs are dullness and depression which develop slowly over several weeks. Along with loss of weight and milk production, a fever appears and the lymph nodes become enlarged. Anemia (low red blood cells) occurs in the latter stages with the appearance of pale membranes in the eye and mouth. Pregnant animals will often abort or experience stillbirths. Although some animals recover, most will die within a short time after symptoms appear.

Diagnosis of trypanosomiasis is based upon observing a combination of symptoms of the individual and other animals in the herd as well as the area where the disease is present. An examination of blood smears of the organism present gives a positive confirmation. Autopsies of animals that have died will show a thin carcass with a paleness to the organs. Often the spleen and lymph nodes will be swollen.

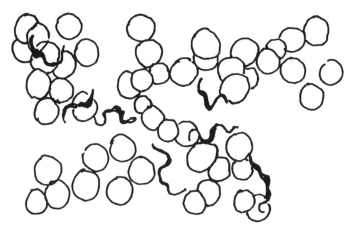

Blood smear with trypanosomes.

In treatment of the disease it is very important to reduce stress and to provide adequate nutrition for sick animals. When using drugs for treatment, it is important to use the proper dosage and recommendations as resistance is a common problem. The following drugs are used most often in treatment programs.

Diminazeve aceturate (Berenil, Ganaseg)
Homidium bromide (Ethidium bromide)
Homidium chloride (Novidium chloride)
Isometamidium chloride (Somorin)
Quinapyramine sulphate (Antrycide)

In addition to using drugs for affected cattle, biological control of the tsetse fly offers great promise in the goal of reducing the occurrence of this serious disease. Since the female mates only once in her lifetime, the release of sterile irradiated males is an effective method to stop the spread of the infective organisms. The release of specific insects that feed on the tsetse fly and traps which attract the fly and kill it are other useful methods of reducing the overall population.

Using cattle that are resistant to the trypanosome protozoa is another method in the program to reduce the level of infection. Such breeds are the humpless West African breeds of N'Dama from Zaire, the Baoule' from the Ivory Coast and Race Locale from the Tongo. Those breeds most affected by this disease are the European and Zebu breeds.

To gain a foothold on this very important disease, a combination of the above will aid in the overall control although elimination is very difficult to ever achieve.

TRICHOMONIASIS

This disease, which is found worldwide, results in infertility and early abortion in cattle. It is caused by *Trichomonas fetus,* a protozoan parasite, and is found only in the reproductive tract of infected animals. Repeat breedings, early abortions, and infections of the uterus are common symptoms of this condition. If pregnancy is maintained until the fifth month, a healthy calf will usually be born. Even though the delivery may be normal, a chronic purulent (yellowish) discharge may be present from the reproductive tract.

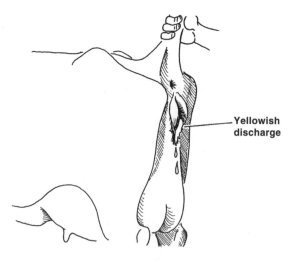

Yellowish discharge

Discharge from vulva.

Removing infected bulls from the herd and using artificial insemination for breeding the cows are the best control methods. A period of sexual rest (no breedings) for 90 days is usually sufficient for the cow to recover from the infection. Bulls, once infected, will remain carriers for life.

Although treatment is available for bulls, it is not performed due to cost and poor rate of cure. If bulls must be used in the breeding program, those under four years of age should be used, as young animals have some natural resistance to the disease.

COCCIDIOSIS

A protozoal parasite, coccidia, lives inside the intestinal cells of infected animals where it can cause serious harm, especially to young animals. The main species of coccidia that affect cattle are *Eimeria zuernii* and *E. bovis*. It is spread directly from animal to animal through contaminated feed and bedding. Where overcrowding is present, coccidia is more of a problem.

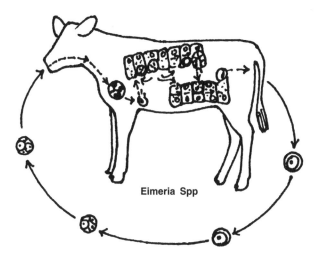

Eimeria Spp

Life cycle of coccidia.

Typical findings of infection are young calves with a foul smelling, dark, watery diarrhea in a crowded, dirty environment. Advanced cases will have clots of blood and mucous in the stool. Without treatment, many animals will lose weight rapidly and die from dehydration. In long standing cases, affected animals will be "poor doers" and never develop normally. Nervous signs may also be present with muscle trembling, convulsions, and a tilting of the neck.

An accurate diagnosis can be made by microscopic examination of the stool along with the typical symptoms found in affected calves. Control of the infection involves the separation of sick animals and good sanitation of the housing area. Not feeding animals on the ground and providing a clean water supply are also very important. Sulfa drugs such as sulfaguanadine are effective as well as ionphores, and amprolium for treating sick animals. For prevention of the disease, drugs such as deccox and amprolium are used. Avoiding pastures that are contaminated with coccidia and over crowding, especially of young animals, are also important in preventing this disease.

Section XVII

Tick Borne Diseases

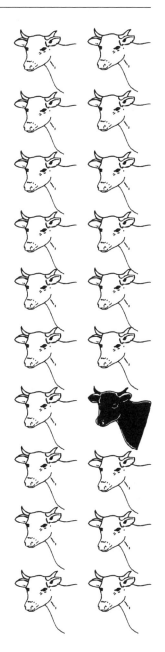

TICK BORNE DISEASES

Ticks are destructive parasites which are very significant economically to the cattle industry. They are present throughout the world but are more widely distributed in the tropical and subtropical countries.

The most serious harm from ticks result from the diseases they transmit to animals. Examples include East Coast Fever, Heartwater, Babesiosis, and Anaplasmosis. Other damage occurs to the hide where the parasites attach in the form of infection and local wounds. Ticks also affect animals by sucking blood from their bodies leaving them in a weaken condition.

There are two groups of ticks; the soft shell, and the hard shell. The soft shell ticks are in the family Argasidae and are mostly found on birds. Hard shell ticks, which are in the family Ixodidae, are the most important to animals. They have a hard covering over most of the upper surface of the male and only a small area of the female.

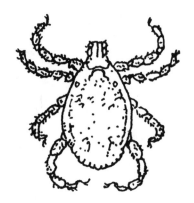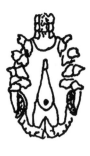

Typical hard shell tick.

All ticks have four pairs of legs and a round body. In the family Ixodidae, the female takes one large blood meal and dies after laying her eggs. The male may feed more than once or sometimes not at all, and ingests only small amounts of blood at a time.

Ticks are grouped by the way in which they undergo development from an egg to a larva (which has 3 pairs of legs), then a nymph, and finally an adult. Most of the life cycle is complete within a year, but some 3 host ticks may live up to a year on each host.

One host ticks remain on the host during its entire life cycle going from the larva to the adult stage. The most common ticks found in this group are *Boophilus sp.*

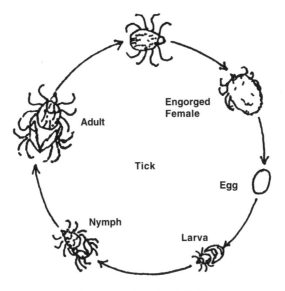

Boophilus (one host tick).

Two host ticks such as the *Rhipicephalus sp.* complete the larva and nymph stage on one host and the adult stage develops on another host.

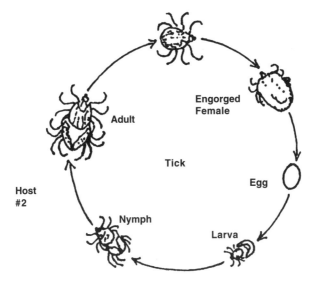

Rhipicephalus (two host tick).

Three host ticks have a different host for each stage of development. Each stage feeds, then drops from the animal to undergo a change to the next form. Finally the engorged female drops to the ground and deposits her eggs, starting another cycle. Species from *Rhipicephalus* and *Amblyomma* are found in this group.

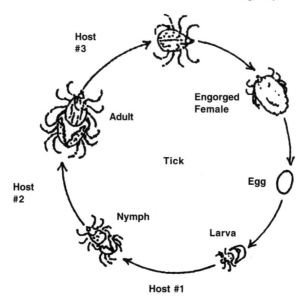

Amblyomma (three host tick).

In most of the species of hard ticks, fertilization occurs while the female is attached to a host. One male may mate with several females. After mating and eating sufficient blood, the female drops to the ground and will lay from 2,000 to 20,000 eggs. She then dies. The male can live much longer than the female and only takes small amounts of blood at a time.

Some common examples of one-host ticks and the diseases they transmit are:

Boophilus decoratus (Blue Tick). Commonly found in South, East and Central Africa. Diseases transmitted are Babesiosis and Anaplasmosis

Boophilus annulatus (North American Cattle Tick). Found in Egypt, Western Asia, and Central America. Transmits Babesiosis.

Boophilus microplus (Blue Cattle Tick). Mainly found in Australia, S.E. Asia, Central and South America, and South Africa. Transmits Babesiosis, Anaplasmosis and Theileriosis.

Examples of two host-ticks and the diseases associated with them are:

Rhipicephalus evertsi (Red-Legged Tick). Found in Central and Southern Africa and transmits East Coast Fever and Babesiosis.
Rhipicephalus bursa. Found in Africa and S.E. Asia. Tranmits Babesiosis, Anaplasmosis, and Theileriosis.
Hyaloam truncatum (African Bont-legged Tick). Transmits sweating sickness in calves and is found in Africa.

Some common three-host ticks are:

Rhipicephalus appenduculatus (Brown Ear Tick). Found in Central, East, and South Africa and transmits East Coast Fever, Corridor Disease, and Babesiosis.
Amblyomma hebracum (Bont or Heartwater Tick). Found in tropical regions and transmits Heartwater.

DISEASES TRANSMITTED BY TICKS

Diseases that are transmitted by ticks differ from many other infections in that young cattle are more resistant or tolerant than older animals to these diseases. When calves are exposed to ticks and the diseases they carry early in life, they experience a mild infection but develop a resistant against further infection. This is similar to a vaccine being given to protect from a future disease. They do remain carriers of the disease for life after being infected, but do not become ill.

In areas where ticks are not present in sufficient numbers to infect calves at an early age, they will be susceptible as adults and may become very sick due to low resistance.

Since tick-born diseases are so important in cattle production, many countries have government programs to aid in tick control. Excellent treatment and control measures can be obtained by writing to the Director of Publications, Food and Agriculture Organization of the United Nations, Via delle Terme di Carocalla, 00100 Rome, Italy.

ANAPLASMOSIS (Gall-Sickness)

Important facts: Can appear very suddenly, or over a long period of time. Causes blood loss, yellow appearance (icterus) and an increased temperature. Found only in ruminants.
Cause: An organism called *Anaplasma marginale* which is a rickettsial agent. It lives in the red blood cells. It is spread by ticks, biting flies, and mechanical means such as needles, dehorning, and castration.

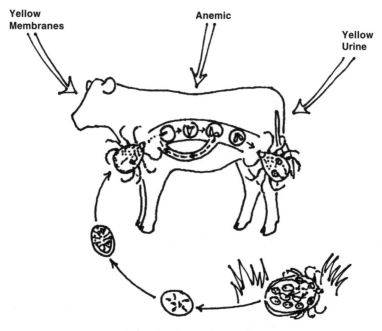

Animal with anaplasmosis.

Symptoms: In calves there is usually a mild infection with little death loss. Older cattle experience a more severe problem with anemia (blood loss) and some deaths (20-50%). Signs include yellow membranes, dark yellow urine, swelling of lymph nodes, depression, and loss of milk production.

Diagnosis: A laboratory examination of a stained blood smear gives the most accurate diagnosis. In areas where Anaplasmosis exists, mature cattle showing anemia without blood in the urine should be suspected of having the disease.

Treatment: Tetracyclines are most often used for treating affected cattle. The long-acting form of the drug is the most effective. Imidocarb dipropionate is another drug that is widely used. If the anemia is severe, blood transfusions and supportive treatment may be necessary.

Control: Spraying or dipping to reduce the level of ticks and other biting insects is done during the vector season. Care should be taken with unclean instruments and needles to avoid transfer of the organism from infected animals to healthy ones. Vaccines are available. Contact local officials for the type of vaccine to be used.

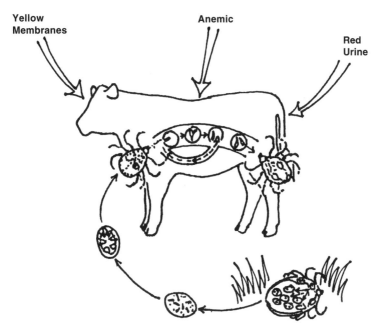

Animal with babesiosis.

BABESIOSIS (Redwater, Piroplasmosis, Tick-Fever)

Important facts: Occurs where ticks are found. Affected animals have a yellowing of the skin, red urine, and are anemic.

Cause: In cattle, the disease is caused by *Babesia bovis* and *Babesia bigemina.* which are protozoal agents. The *Boophilus sp* is the major tick vector, but biting flies and other ticks can also transmit the disease.

Symptoms: Animals may become sick very quickly or over a long period of time. Young animals are affected more with this disease. Fever up to 107 degrees F (42 degrees C) may occur followed by loss of appetite and depression. The skin and membranes may turn yellow and the urine may be reddish.

Diagnosis: Affected animals with a high fever, anemia, yellow membranes, and red urine in a tick infested area is diagnostic for babesiosis. Positive identification is made by examination of a blood smear which shows the organisms.

Treatment: The infection responds well if treated early in the course of the disease. In long standing cases, blood transfusions and supportive therapy may be necessary. Quinuronium sulfate (Pirevan) is an older drug that is still used with success. Newer therapy includes medications such as phenamidine isethionate, amicarbalide de-isethionate (Diampron), diminazene aceturate (Berenil), and imidocarb dipropionate (Imizol). In cattle that have been treated, the parasites are completely eliminated from the blood and no immunity results; therefore the protozoan can infect the animal again.

Control: One effective control method is to eliminate the tick vectors by use of sprays and dips. However, this is not often economically possible. Vaccines are available in certain areas. They contain weak strains of the babesia parasite. Another method of control is by premunition: the animals are exposed slowly to the disease organism by either using weak vaccines or using low amounts of drugs to weaken the organism, thereby giving the animal a chance to build its own immunity.

TICK PARALYSIS

Important facts: A sudden paralysis starting in the rear of the animal and moving forward, in tick infested areas. Affects most animals as well as man.

Cause: A nerve toxin released from a tick attached to the body.

Symptoms: A weakness which begins in the rear legs and moves toward the head. Total paralysis can develop within a few hours and results in death when the muscles of respiration are affected.

Diagnosis: Typical symptoms in areas where ticks are found in the absence of other signs.

Treatment: Removal of the tick either manually or by dips or sprays results in almost immediate improvement.

Control: Avoiding tick-infested areas and using dips and sprays to eliminate the ticks.

Section XVIII

Parasitic Diseases

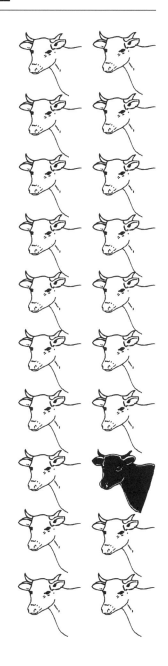

PARASITES

Small organisms that live off other animals (hosts) are called parasites. Many different types exist: small and large, internal and external, beneficial and harmful.

In cattle, the concern is mostly with the parasites that are found on the surface of the body (ectoparasites) and those found inside the body (internal parasites).

ECTOPARASITES

These parasites live on the surfface of their host and cause irritation to the animal as well as damage to the skin and hair, resulting in wounds which lead to infection. The most common are ticks, flies, lice, and mites.

Mites: These are small tick-like organisms that have four pairs of legs. They are much smaller than ticks. In cattle they produce various types of mange which damage the skin and cause inflammation by their burrowing action. The two most important mites in cattle are the demodectic and scarcoptic.

Demodectic mange is caused by *Demodex bovis.*

Demodectic mite life cycle.

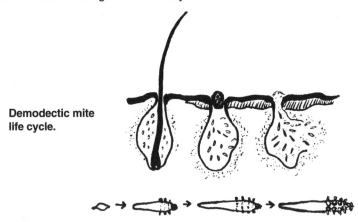

The demodex mite is found in the follicle of the hair and is a normal occurrence in healthy skin. In some animals the mite multiplies at a greater than normal rate and causes the lesions (sores), associated with demodectic manage. It occurs most frequently around the eyelids, vulva or scrotum. Although the mites grow very slowly, and the damage to the skin can be slight at first, wounds and infection may result from the irritation caused as the mites multiply. They are diagnosed by microscopic examination of skin scrapings. Treatments in-

144

clude dips with 2% rotenone preparations in oil and repeated injections of ivermectin at 2-4 week intervals. A complete cure is very difficult to obtain.

Sarcoptic mange is caused by *Sarcoptes scabei.*

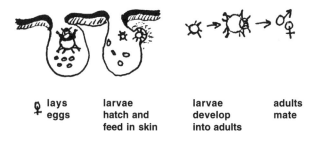

♀ lays	larvae	larvae	adults
eggs	hatch and	develop	mate
	feed in skin	into adults	

Scabies mite life cycle.

This is a very contagious mite which is spread by direct contact with other animals. It also lives deep in the skin and causes an intense itching and inflammation of the skin resulting in sores from the animal rubbing and scratching. Diagnosis is by finding the mite from skin scrapings with a microscope. The most effective treatment is the use of ivermectin given at 2-4 week intervals until the mites are killed. Other methods of treating include dips using gammexane (lindane), lime sulphur (2% calcium polysulphide), coumaphos (Co-Ral), and 5% solution toxaphene.

FLIES AND THEIR IMPORTANCE TO CATTLE

Although flies are not thought of as a serious problem, they are responsible for high economic losses in many areas of the world. Some of the more important flies associated with cattle are the house, face, deer, stable and horsefly. The warble and screw worm fly are also important because of the damage they do to the hide and skin of cattle. In order to control flies, it is important to identify the type of fly, its behavior and life cycle.

HOUSE FLY

The common house fly is normally found where humans and animals live. It is gray in color, with four dark stripes running down its back, and the face is a pale, straw color. The house fly feeds with a swabbing motion of its mouth parts and does not suck blood. It is close to 1/4 inch (6 mm) in size. While we generally think of house flies as carriers of disease, they also disturb cattle with their feeding practices. During hot, sunny days they are most active.

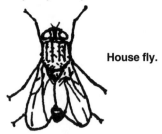

House fly.

House flies start their activity during the first warm months when they begin to lay eggs in manure and garbage. There may be up to four batches of eggs (100-150 per laying) deposited by the female. After 24 hours, the eggs hatch into maggots or larvae. After seven days, the larvae are fully grown at which time they pupate. In one more week, adult flies emerge and start to lay eggs in another two weeks. In warm weather, the cycle may be shorter. The maggots or pupae can over winter in cool climates or the adults may survive in heated buildings.

STABLE FLY

In appearance and size, the stable fly is similar to the house fly. It has a stronger, well developed, black penetrating-sucking mouth part.

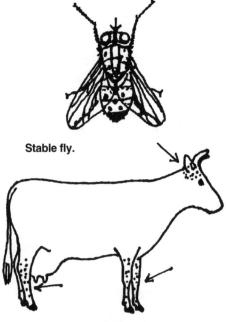

Stable fly.

In addition, the back and abdomen have large dark spots. When not feeding on cattle, it prefers to rest in shaded areas on trees or buildings. When cattle are grazing, they are bothered more by the stable fly than when at rest. The ears and legs are the areas most affected during feeding which is only during the daylight hours. When observed feeding on the animal, they are generally facing upwards.

Eggs from the stable fly are laid in manure and rotting vegetation. Only after the female has consumed three blood meals does she start the egg laying process. This may be as soon as 10 days after the fly emerges from the pupae. About 30 days is required for the complete cycle from egg to adult. Several generations may occur during the year. In cool climates, the maggots and pupae remain in piles of manure.

FACE FLY

In appearance and size the face fly is very similar to the house fly and identification is usually made by where it is found feeding on the cow. The face and head area is where large numbers may be found, especially around the eyes and mouth. Eye problems are often blamed on the face fly as it may be a carrier of the pink eye organism. In warm weather it usually rests in the sunlight close to where animals are found.

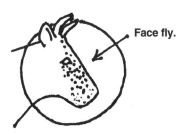

Face fly.

The life cycle of the face fly is very similar to the house fly except the female is capable of producing as many as 1500 eggs in her life. Fresh manure is where the eggs are laid and develop. Adults often over winter in warm buildings.

DEER FLY

This fly is larger than the house fly and its body is yellow with brown stripes. It has a piercing-sucking mouth part and the wings have a brown band. They are aggressive flies and may cause bleeding wounds by their feeding behavior. They are more active on warm days but only during the daylight hours.

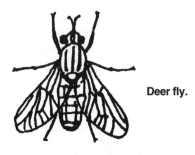

Deer fly.

Eggs from the deer fly are attached to vegetation in moist areas. After hatching, the larva migrate to the soil where they stay for one or more winters, finally emerging as pupae and then maturing into adults.

HORN FLY

This is a dark gray fly about one-half the size of the house fly measuring a little more than 1/8 inch (3 mm), and it has piercing-sucking mouth parts. It feeds on cattle both day and night, only leaving to lay eggs. They can be found feeding along the horns, behind the neck and on the withers. They are unlike the stable fly in that they feed facing downwards. In warm weather, they are found more on the belly or around the udder. Adults live about three weeks and survive only on blood meals.

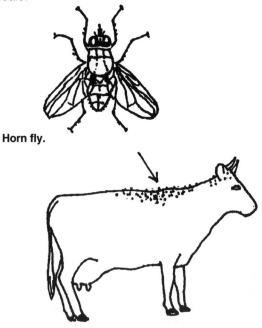

Horn fly.

Eggs are laid in fresh cow manure where they hatch in less than a day. Here the larvae develop another five days and pupate. After five days, adults emerge and within 2-3 hours begin feeding. After the third day, females can begin laying eggs. Only a small number of eggs, approximately 20, are produced during the short three week adult life.

HORSE FLY

This is the largest of the flies. It can cause a painful bite from its large piercing-sucking mouth parts. In addition to its size, it can be recognized by the large round eyes and the loud buzzing sound made while in flight. Males only feed on flowers and are not a threat to livestock. Only a few females attack at any one time and feeding is usually limited to the back of the animal. They are only active during the day and prefer warm sunny periods.

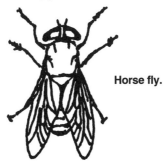

Horse fly.

The life cycle is similar to the deer fly where the eggs are found in moist areas, and the larvae can live for a long period before completing their life cycle.

CONTROL OF FLIES

Sanitation is a must to keep the fly populations low, especially around the barn where cattle are concentrated. Anywhere manure accumulates, flies will breed and multiply, therefore cattle should be pastured away from milking and handling facilities as much as possible.

For treating the individual animals, several options are available. Before using any chemicals for fly control, be sure to read the instructions carefully to avoid contamination of the meat and milk. Products are manufactured to be used as powders, sprays, fogs, and back rubbers. Some of the more common ones are: Coumaphos (CO-RAL), Crotoxyphos (Ciodrin), Dichlorvos (Vapona), Pyrethrins and Stirofos (Rabon).

Some products are to be used only in the milking barns and livestock should not be present when applying the chemicals. Manufacturers have also developed insecticides to be mixed in the feed to control flies. The agent passes through the digestive tract and leaves no residue in the meat or milk. Another novel way is to mix insecticides in paint or whitewash and apply it to the walls of barns to repel flies.

In summary, flies are an important insect to control in a cattle operation. They contribute to a loss of weight and milk production by their blood sucking and irritation. Many methods are used to reduce the overall fly population, but among the most important is good sanitation especially in and around the barn and milking areas.

CATTLE GRUB WORM (Warble fly, Heel fly)

Infestation with the warble fly or cattle grub is called hypodermosis. In the Northern Hemisphere, flies of the genus *Hypoderma* are the most important while in the Southern Hemisphere, the Dermatobia species is seen more frequently.

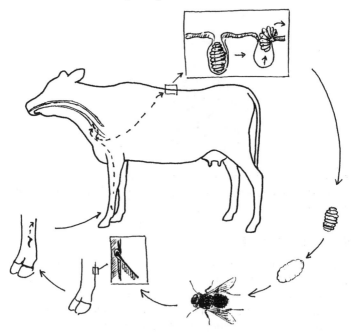

Hypoderma cycle.

Hypoderma species

This cattle grub occurs in the Northern Hemisphere between 25 and 60 degrees latitude in North America, Europe, Africa, and Asia. The adult Hypoderma (heel flies) attach their eggs on the hair of cattle's lower legs. In 3 to 7 days, the eggs hatch and the first-stage larva penetrate the skin. They travel throughout the body locating in two areas depending on the species. *Hypoderma lineatum* species find their way to the esophageal wall while *Hypoderma bovis* are found in the area of the spinal canal. They stay here for 2 to 4 months.

In early winter, the larvae begin to migrate again. This time they end up under the skin on the back where they make a breathing hole in the skin. Here they undergo two molts which last 4 to 6 weeks. Then the larvae emerge from the hole and drop to the ground and pupate. In 1 to 3 months, adult flies hatch from the larvae, completing the life cycle which takes about one year. Adults live less than one week and do not feed during their brief Life, but do accomplish the important task of laying eggs to begin the cycle again.

When cattle are observed on warm sunny days running through the pasture with their tails high in the air, it is usually in response to attacks by heel flies.

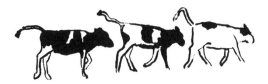

Cattle running from heel flies.

Normal feeding is often interrupted by the flies, resulting in a weight loss. Once the larvae enter the body, visible results of their presence is not seen until they emerge on the back through a breathing hole. In some instances, animals will experience bloat or swallowing problems from their presence in the esophageal tissue. Soreness in the back and rarely paralysis may also occur while the larvae are in the tissue around the spinal canal. Holes in the skin from the presence of the grubs cause a marked reduction of the value of the hide.

Treatment of the grubs can be accomplished with various insecticides. Pour-on treatments of ivermectin, trichlorfon, coumaphos, famphur, fenthion, and phosmet should be applied evenly along the midline of the back. When using a 20% solution of fenthion, it should be applied in a single spot on the back. Sprays containing coumaphous or phosmet are also effective as well as the injectable form of ivermectin. The treatments should be used carefully as they may cause stress in the animals. Organophosphates and ivermectin are prohibited in milking dairy cattle because residues are present for long periods of time in the milk. Ectoline (Fibronil) is a newer pour-on that is very effective but can be used only in non-lactating cattle. Withdrawal times should be observed very carefully with any treatment.

As soon as possible after the end of the heel fly season, affected cattle should be treated. Later treatment should not be given earlier than 8 to 12 weeks before the grubs make their appearance in the back. This is to avoid adverse reactions that may occur if migratory larvae are killed in the body.

When pour-on or injectable drugs are not available or approved, rotenone may be used to control the grubs. To be effective, the drug must be worked into the breathing holes to make contact with the larvae. If applied in the correct manner, over 90% of the grubs will be killed. Manual extraction of the grubs can also be performed, however, a serious reaction may result in the animal if the larvae are crushed within their cysts.

Dermatopia species

The most common name for this cattle grub is the Tropical Warble Fly or Torsalo. Its distribution is in warmer climates especially in Central and South America. Although it occurs in many species, as well as man, cattle and dogs are affected the most.

Living only an average of four days, the small adult fly attaches its eggs to different types of insects (mostly flies and mosquitoes) which transport them to the host animal while they are feeding. After hatching, the larvae migrate through the body for 1 to 2 months, finally coming to rest in the skin where the warble forms a breathing hole. After maturing, the larvae emerge through the hole and drop to the ground where they pupate and develop into adult flies. The life cycle is complete in 3 to 4 months.

During the time the larval migration is occurring in the body there may be local pain and inflammation in the host animal, resulting in loss of weight and milk production. The hide also is decreased in value due to the damage from the breathing holes.

The treatment and control is by sprays, dips, pour-on's, and injections. Organophosphates such as dichlorvos and fenthion are commonly used. Ivermectin may be used as an injectable or pour-on.

SCREWWORM INFESTATION

Larvae from the screwworm fly, *Cochliomyia hominivorax*, is a serious problem in cattle throughout Central and South America. When the screwworm fly, also known as the blowfly, lays her eggs in wounds, cuts, bites, naval cords, and other sites, a very destructive larvae develops. Death of the affected animal may occur unless the larvae are controlled.

The cycle begins when the female screwworm fly deposits from 200 to 400 eggs in a broken area of the skin. Within one day the eggs hatch into the larval stage. In the process of feeding, the developing parasite can cause serious damage to the surrounding tissue. Within 5 to 7

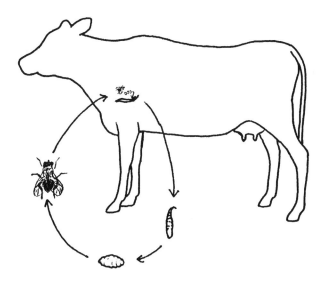

Cochliomyia cycle.

days, the larvae leave the wound, drop to the ground, and burrow into the soil to pupate. After one week to two months, the adults hatch and mate when 3 to 4 days old. In one week the females mate one time and begin to lay eggs, completing the life cycle.

To control the screwworm, a smear containing lindane or ronnel is applied directly to the affected site. A thin layer may be applied around fresh wounds to prevent the occurrence of infestation. Sprays, dust, and foam preparations are also used to control and treat the larval stage. Ivermectin given as an injection will also kill the larvae and prevent reinfestation for up to two weeks.

Elimination of the flies is an effective way to control screwworms. The two major methods used are sterile males and insecticides. Since the female fly only mates once, introducing male flies that have been sterilized by irradiation to breed the females is an effective method to reduce the fly population. Another efficient tool is to use a screwworm attractant with an insecticide to kill the flies.

PEDICULOSIS (Louse Infestation, Lice)

Lice are grouped as either sucking or biting insect. These insects affect cattle and other mammals. They are fairly host specific and cannot complete a life cycle except on the animal they are adapted to. They are more of a problem in the cooler months of the year.

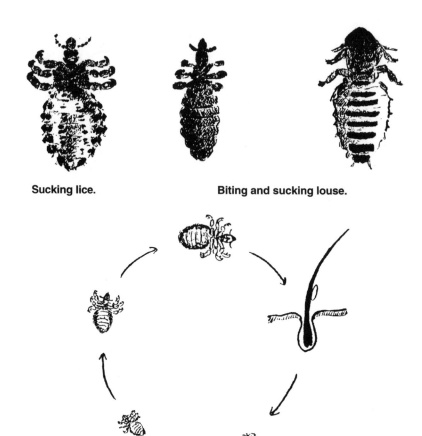

Sucking lice.   Biting and sucking louse.

Life cycle of a sucking louse.

Transmission of the small wingless insects requires direct contact with other animals. Their three pairs of legs are developed to cling tightly to the hair as they feed or suck blood from their host. Eggs laid from adults are sticky and attach to the hair. From 3 to 4 weeks are required to complete a generation.

An intense itching sensation results from the biting and sucking action of the lice. In severe cases, hair loss occurs and open wounds may result from the rubbing. Heavy infestation with sucking lice may result in anemia and loss of body weight and milk production.

Effective treatment of lice requires the use of the correct insecticide, however, many products are not allowed because of possible residues in the meat or milk. If local regulations allow, the following may be used in lactating dairy animals. Compounds containing crotoxyphos, crotoxyphos plus dichlorvos, and permethrin. Coumaphos, fenvalerate, and stirofos are also effective. Injectable ivermectin is very reliable for controlling sucking lice, but it is not approved for use for cattle in milk production.

INTERNAL PARASITES

Stomach worms

Three major groups of parasites that live in the stomach of cattle are *Haemonchus placei* (barber's pole worm), *Ostertgia ostertagi* (brown stomach worm), and *Trichostrongylus axei* (small stomach worm).

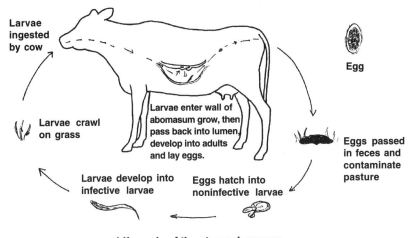

Life cycle of the stomach worms.

The life cycle of the three worms is similar. Adults live in the digestive tract and lay eggs which are passed in the manure. Infective larvae then hatch and are ingested up by the animal while grazing, and develop into adults. In warm climates, the entire process may be completed in 2 to 4 weeks. The larvae however, remain dormant for long periods of time in cooler environments.

As the ingested larvae and adults feed in the stomach, they cause damage by their blood sucking ability and irritation to the stomach wall. Also the normal pH in the abomasum (4th stomach)is altered by the presence of the larvae which can result in severe diarrhea and loss of protein absorption.

Animals affected with ostertagia and trichostrongylus show signs of watery diarrhea which is worse in the young. In haemonchosis infection, there is usually no diarrhea. Anemia is common with all three parasites. A common finding resulting from the anemia and diarrhea is a swelling under the jaw (bottle jaw). Affected animals also experience weight loss, rough hair coat, and loss of appetite.

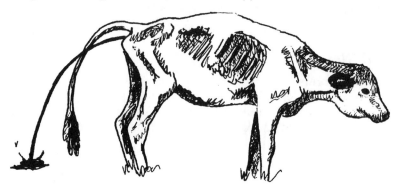

Animal affected with stomach worms.

Intestinal worms

In the first 10 to 20 feet of the small intestine, several species of Cooperia (bankrupt worm) occur. It is a small worm that causes irritation to the lining of the intestine, but it does not suck blood. The most common sign of infection is diarrhea with weight loss but no anemia.

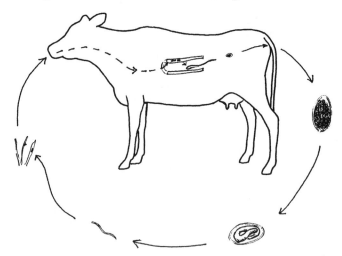

Life cycle of cooperia spp.

Another worm commonly found in the first few feet of the intestines is *Bunostomum phlebotomum* (cattle hookworm). An interesting fact with this parasite is its ability to enter the body through skin penetration as well as via the mouth during feeding. In addition to causing damage to the lining of the gut wall, it also causes anemia from its feeding action.

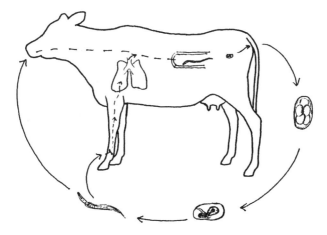

Life cycle of bunostomum spp.

Strongyloides papillosus, the intestinal threadworm, is commonly found lower in the digestive tract. Only female worms are parasitic to the animal. Entry into the body is either by penetration through the skin or by ingestion. Signs relating to infection is usually a slight diarrhea, and associated loss of weight.

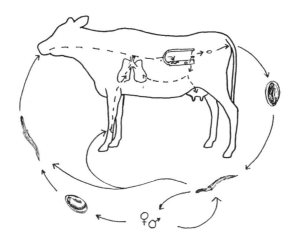

Strongyloides life cycle.

A parasite that seems to appear more often after a heavy rain storm is *Nematodirus helvetianus* (thin-necked intestinal worm). The eggs develop slowly, containing the infective larval stage of the worm. The presence of water causes the eggs to hatch very rapidly releasing the larvae to be released in large numbers in grazing areas. Clinical signs noted with nematodirus are relatively mild. Diarrhea and loss of appetite are the main symptoms.

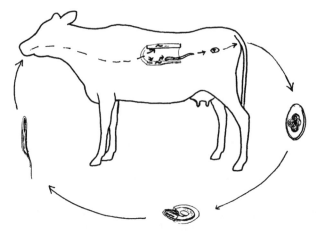

Nematodirus life cycle.

One of the larger adult worms is *Toxocara vitulurum*. It is found mainly in the small intestine of young calves. Adults develop a resistance to the parasite, although the infective larvae is passed to the calf through the colostrum. A heavy infection can be serious in the young animal.

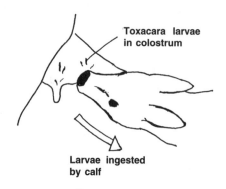

Toxacara larvae in colostrum

Larvae ingested by calf

Toxocara cycle.

Young animals suffer diarrhea and weight loss from *Oesophagostomum radiatum* (nodular worm), while adults have problems with intestinal motility due to nodules caused by the parasite. The common name, nodular worm, relates to the reaction of the tissue from the migration of the larvae. In severe cases, the intestinal tract may be obstructed or turned in on itself (intussusception) due to the irritation.

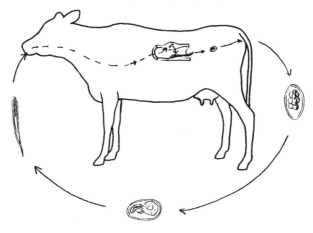

Oesophagostomum life cycle.

In young calves and yearlings, *Trichuris species* (cattle whipworm), can cause clinical signs such as anemia and weight loss if a large number of eggs are present on the farm. However, with general sanitation measures, it is seldom a problem.

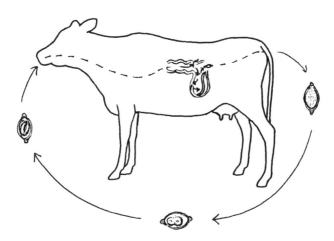

Trichuris life cycle.

159

TAPEWORM

A small mite is part of the life cycle of the tapeworm, *Moniezia benedeni,* which occurs primarily in young calves. The eggs pass from the animal and are ingested by the mite, where the infective stage develops. The small mites are then eaten by the animal while grazing, completing the life cycle. Although seldom a concern in calves, the digestive process may be slowed due to the presence of the worms.

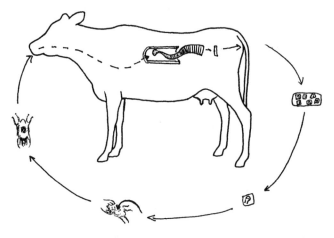

Moniezia life cycle.

DIAGNOSIS OF PARASITES FOUND IN THE INTESTINAL TRACT

In many cases the diagnosis of intestinal parasites can be made on the basis of the signs present, the season and the grazing history. The infection can be verified by examination of the feces under a microscope.

A simple test solution can be made by preparing a concentrated sugar and water mixture. A small amount of manure is mixed into the solution and placed in a test tube to set for 15 to 20 minutes. If worm eggs are present in the stool, they will float to the top of the mixture. A drop from the top of the tube is transferred to a glass slide and examined under the microscope for the presence of worm eggs.

An autopsy of an animal that has died is also a valuable means of identifying what parasites are present in the herd and the severity of an infection.

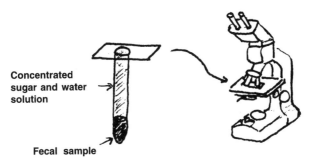

Concentrated sugar and water solution →

Fecal sample →

Examination for worm eggs.

CONTROL AND TREATMENT OF INTESTINAL PARASITES

Many drugs are available to treat worms found in the intestinal tract. In choosing a suitable product, the availability, ease of administration, and effectiveness should be considered. Also, the safety, and length of residue in the meat and milk is very important especially in dairy animals producing milk.

The following are a list of the most commonly used medicines for treating intestinal worms.

Ivermectin: Ivomec.
Benzimidazoles: Thiabendazole, Fenbendezole, Mebendazole, Oxfendazole, Mebendazole, Aldendazole.
Imidazathiazoles: Levamisole, Tramisol.
Organophosphates: Baymix, Halox, Loxan
Phenothiazine: Tefenco, Febantel.
Morantel Tartorate: Rumatel, Nemater.
Lead arsenate
Niclosamide

The above products come in a variety of forms, including injections, sprays, dips, pour-on', gels, pastes, boluses, drenches, and premixes for the feed. It is very important to follow the manufacturers recommendations for the dosage and withdrawal guidelines.

Controlling future infections of intestinal worms is of primary concern. We should be careful to prevent the heavy build-up egg populations in the pasture and to encourage the development of immunity and resistance in the cattle. To accomplish this, a knowledge of the life cycle of the parasites is necessary together with the feeding habits

161

of the animals. Young stock are usually affected more severely and should be monitored closely during their growing period. Rotation of the herd to clean feeding areas is a way to reduce exposure during critical periods as well as removal of manure and taking care that the feed and water are not contaminated.

LUNGWORM INFECTION

A condition involving the respiratory tract which can be severe in young animals is caused by *Dictyocaulus viviparus*. The most common signs are coughing with rapid and shallow breathing, especially after exercise. Affected adults can experience a loss of both weight and milk production with a heavy infection.

The life cycle is direct, therefore the eggs are passed in the manure, develop into larva, and are ingested by the cow. Inside the digestive tract they pass through the gut and are carried by the blood system to the lungs, where they become adults ready to lay eggs again.

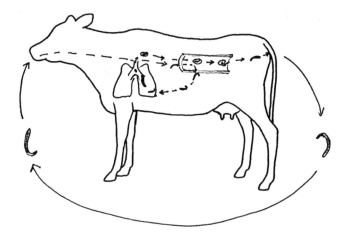

Lungworm life cycle.

A diagnosis is usually made by observation of signs, autopsy, and finding the larvae in a microscopic examination. A modification of the Baermann technique to examine the feces is usually effective in finding the larvae. A sample of the manure is wrapped in tissue paper or cheese cloth, suspended in a beaker of water, and allowed to set for 4 or more hours. The larvae will generally be found in the bottom of the solution, and can be identified by use of a microscope.

Treatment of lungworms is accomplished with several different drugs. Levamisole, ivermectin, and products from the benzimidazole

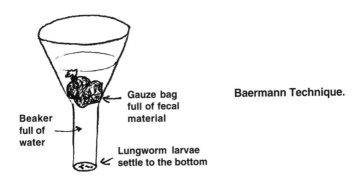

Gauze bag
full of fecal
material

Beaker
full of
water

Lungworm larvae
settle to the bottom

Baermann Technique.

group (fenbendazole, oxfendazole, and albendazole) are effective against all stages of the parasite.

Control by pasture rotation alone is not reliable. Calves should not be allowed to graze on areas known to be infected with lungworms, as their resistance is very low. In general, adult animals will have immunity to the worms unless there is a heavy infection. Using a worming program with pasture rotation has shown to give good control. A program where cattle are treated at 3 and 8 weeks after entering the grazing area is effective in reducing the problem.

LIVER FLUKE INFECTION

The most important cause of liver disease in cattle is caused by a trematode called *Fasciola hepatica,* also known as the common liver fluke. It is very common in warm tropical areas of the world.

The development of the liver fluke requires wet areas and an intermediate host to complete the life cycle. As the eggs pass in the manure, they hatch in a moist area, and enter a water snail (intermediate host) where further development takes place. After 1 to 2 months, the second stage emerge from the snail and attach to vegetation in wet areas where they form a cyst around themselves. At this stage they are infective and once eaten by a grazing animal, they pass through the gut wall and penetrate the liver. After entering the bile ducts, they mature into adults, and start to produce eggs.

Although rarely fatal in cattle, serious damage can occur to the liver and bile duct. In heavy infections animals can become anemic, loose weight, and experience loss in meat and milk production.

An accurate diagnosis of liver flukes is based on clinical signs, a history of grazing in wet areas with heavy snail populations, and finding the fluke eggs with microscopic examination of the feces. The eggs are heavy and will sink to the bottom of the testing solution,

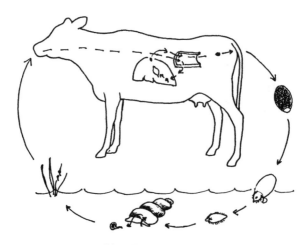

Liver fluke life cycle.

therefore the sediment should be examined when making a diagnosis. Since egg production varies even in a heavy infection, several tests may be required to demonstrate the eggs.

In controlling liver flukes, it is important to remember the role of the water snail in the life cycle. Drugs can be used against the flukes in the animal, but measures must also be taken to reduce the intermediate host, the snail.

The most commonly used drugs against liver flukes are albendazole and clorsulon. Other drugs are rafoxanide, nitroxynil, closantel, tricla-bendazole, and netobimin.

To control the water snail, the most common method is to drain wet marshy areas where the snail lives. Copper compounds, sodium pentachlorphenate, and trifenmorph are commonly used to reduce the snails if drainage is not possible. Fencing off marshy areas is another method of keeping cattle from grazing where snails are located.

Section **XIX**

Non Infectious Diseases

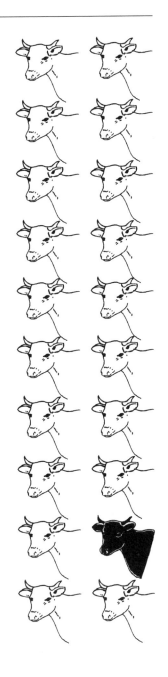

NON-INFECTIOUS CONDITIONS

CHOKE

Choke occurs when a foreign object lodges in the throat or esophagus (food tube). The most common foods that cause choking are be round items such as apples, potatoes, or beets. An affected animal is usually seen with its neck stretched out, and mouth open. Drooling is usually present and breathing may be labored if bloating is present.

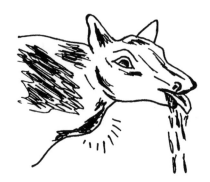

Choke in a cow.

To relieve the choke, a mouth gag must be placed in the cow's mouth to allow passage of a hand or instrument down into the throat. In some cases the object can be removed with the hand or a wire loop. If this is not possible, a stiff stomach tube may be used to push the obstruction into the stomach. This may cause a tear of the esophagus, which could be fatal, so must be performed with care.

HARDWARE DISEASE

This is a condition in which small pieces of wire or metal that have been eaten with grass or hay lodge in the second stomach (reticulum, honeycomb). During the movement of the stomach during digestion, the objects may penetrate through the wall and enter the heart sac causing an infection around the heart.

The signs are depression, loss of milk production, and weight loss. The back may be arched along with a reluctance to move due to pain. A grunt may be heard as the animal moves. Often the body temperature is elevated.

Treatment involves the use of a magnet administered orally in the hope to pull the metal away from the heart. Antibiotics should also be given to fight infection. Surgery can be performed in valuable animals.

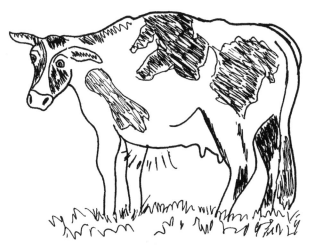

Hardware Disease
Cow with an arched back, pain in chest.

WATERBELLY (Urinary stones)

This is usually seen in castrated males. It results when small stones (calculi, mineral stones) form in the bladder and become lodged in the tube (urethra) that carries urine to the penis. Urine cannot escape and backs up in the bladder causing it to rupture.

The first signs of a urinary blockage will be a discomfort of the animal along with constantly getting up or lying down. The tail may be up in the air or twisting from side to side as attempts are made to urinate. Once the bladder ruptures, dullness and depression set in. A swelling will soon follow as urine accumulates under the skin of the belly or within the abdominal cavity.

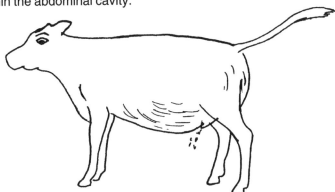

Steer with a water belly.

Early treatment is necessary to save the life of the animal. A surgical incision above the scrotum is made to redirect the flow of urine away from the penis. Making sure plenty of water is available and providing the correct mineral balance helps to prevent this condition.

VAGINAL AND RECTAL PROLAPSE

This condition often occurs before or after calving. The vaginal (birth canal) will often evert due to swelling or straining from the cow. A complication from the vaginal eversion may be a urinary blockage. A rectal prolapse may follow due to the cow pushing from the irritation of the prolapsed vagina or from trying to urinate.

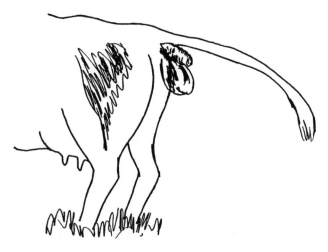

Prolapsed vagina and rectum.

Both conditions require immediate attention and a trained person, as an injection must be given to relieve the straining and pain. The tissues are then inverted back into the animal and sutures placed to prevent recurrence.

LAMENESS

The most common causes of non-infectious lameness in cattle are abscesses in the hoof wall, puncture wounds in the foot, and inflammation (arthritis) in the joints of the lower leg.

When an abscess involves the foot, it is usually located within the hoof wall. A puncture wound is the most common cause. Very little swelling occurs, but the foot is very sore and tender. To treat the con-

168

dition, the cow must be restrained with ropes and the area of the abscess located and drained. Antibiotics are packed in the area, and the foot is wrapped until healing takes place.

Puncture wounds to the foot are fairly common and may involve a nail, sharp stone, or piece of wire. Once the problem is located, the object is removed, the area cleaned and antibiotics applied to the wound. A bandage around the injured area is helpful until it heals

Arthritis usually occurs following an injury or puncture wound to a joint. It may be noted as a local swelling or tenderness. Treatment is directed at resting the joint and applying heat to reduce the swelling. A cure may not be possible if the joint damage is severe.

LAMINITIS (Founder)

This is a condition that occurs when the animal has a rapid change of feed, usually from a high fiber to a high energy diet such as grain or protein. The front feet usually become very painful due to swelling in the hoof area. After the initial attack, the hoofs become elongated from a rapid growth rate stimulated from the inflammation in the hoof wall. Treatment is aimed at relieving the pain and frequent hoof trimming.

BLOAT

When gas accumulates in the rumen, or paunch, and the animal cannot get rid of it, a condition called bloat occurs. This problem has many causes but the most common are choke, paralysis of the stomach muscles, and rapid ingestion of feeds that form gas.

The most obvious symptom of bloat is a swelling on the left side of the animal where the rumen is located. Other signs are drooling, difficult breathing, mouth open, and a reluctance to move. If the bloat is not relieved, the animal will eventually lie down and die because the swelling interferes with the ability to breathe.

When an animal is having trouble breathing, it is considered an emergency. The gas must be relieved immediately! The most effective way is to puncture the rumen with a sharp knife, scissors, or trochar. The point of puncture is on the left side at a point halfway between the last rib and the point of the hip and the same distance down from the back. When using a knife or scissors, a hollow tube or bamboo can be placed in the hole to allow the gas to escape. A trochar has a hollow tube around the sharp point which can be left in place to vent the gas.

One type of bloat which is called "frothy bloat" is very difficult to treat. It occurs when the gas is trapped in bubbles which do not pass easily through a stomach tube or trocar. The only solution is to use

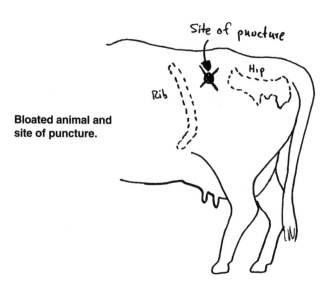

Bloated animal and site of puncture.

medications to dissolve the air bubbles. Vegetable oils such as peanut, soybean, or corn are very helpful. Usually a pint is given either by stomach tube or directly into the rumen if a tube is in place. Cream from milk is also useful in an emergency as well as household detergents mixed with water.

After treating the bloat, the animal should be observed carefully for recurrence of signs. The puncture wound should be treated to avoid screwworms and local infection.

LIGHTNING STRIKE

When one or more cattle are suddenly found dead after a severe storm lying under a tree or on top of a hill, one should be very suspicious of death by lightning. There may also be scorch marks on trees or along the ground, or burns on the animal's hair. A post mortem examination is usually not very diagnostic.

SNAKEBITE

In tropical countries, snakebite is a common occurrence in animals. They are usually bit on the face or legs while grazing. Puncture marks in these areas with swelling and inflammation is diagnostic for snakebite. Depending on the type of snake and amount of venom injected, the symptoms can be mild to severe. Treatment involves cleaning the wound, rest, antibiotics, and anti-inflammatory drugs.

POISONINGS FROM TOXIC SUBSTANCES.

Animals are often affected by toxic agents which are found in plants, chemicals, and certain minerals. Common symptoms may range from increased excitability, dullness, liver damage, salivation, convulsions, and skin blistering. Since the signs vary, it is difficult to make a diagnosis in many cases. If a laboratory is available, samples such as blood, feces, or autopsy tissues may assist in determining the cause of a suspected poisoning.

In tropical areas, plant poisoning is fairly common because the high temperatures and humidity favor the growth of many toxic plants. Also, in arid climates, cattle often eat harmful toxic plants, which they would otherwise avoid, due to hunger. It should be remembered that young animals are more susceptible to toxins.

Treatment for most plant poisonings is to relieve the symptoms, since very few specific antidotes exist. Medications are given to absorb the harmful substances or to deactivate them. Charcoals, limewater, and alum help to prevent poisons from entering the blood stream, while lubricants, such as linseed or mineral oil, reduce intestinal irritation and help to speed the removal of the toxic agents from the body. Convulsions are treated with depressants (barbiturates) while depressed animals can be given stimulants. Avoiding grazing areas where toxic plants are found and clipping pastures are important in prevention program.

Arsenic, copper, nitrates, and lead are common substances that cause damage to animals.

Arsenic, which is used in dips and sprays, causes severe intestinal irritation leading to colic, pain, and diarrhea. Sodium thiosulphate (60-120gm) given as a drench may give some relief as a treatment. Dimercaprol (BAL) is a specific antidote which is given as an injection.

Poisoning from copper usually results from improper supplementation or from accidental spraying of cattle feeds with copper salts. Symptoms occur after long periods of exposure and include yellow skin, pain, and bloody urine. No specific treatment is available other than avoidance of the source.

Lead poisoning can cause blindness, nervous signs, depression, abdominal pain, constipation and even death. Common sources of lead are old paint, batteries, and discarded oil. Magnesium sulfate (epsom salts) given by mouth can be used to remove lead from the digestive tract. A drug called calcium disodium edetate (CaEDTA) given in the vein helps to draw the lead from the body tissues to be excreted in the urine.

During periods of low rainfall or little sunlight and after heavy applications of fertilizer, plants often accumulate large amounts of nitrates.

When ingested by cattle, a condition known as nitrate poisoning occurs. Signs include panting, gasping, bloat, and depression due to a chemical reaction which prevents oxygen from being carried in the blood. Pregnant animals that recover may abort. Death often follows in a few hours without treatment in severe cases. Intravenous administration of 2% methylene blue is a specific antidote to nitrate poisoning. Mineral oil may also be given to reduce irritation to the intestines.

Creosote compounds, such as diesel and paraffin products, can cause a variety of symptoms when ingested. Low levels of creosote will cause a poor haircoat and reduced growth, while higher amounts will result in depression, abdominal pain, and nervous signs. No specific treatment is available.

Insecticides are usually divided into two main groups which cause poisoning. They are chlorinated hydrocarbons and organophosphates. Common agents which contain chlorinated hydrocarbons are DDT, BHC, and Dieldrin. Symptoms include excitability and muscle spasms. Treatment is limited to controlling the nervous signs. Organophosphates occur in many insecticides such as fly repellents, cattle wormers, and crop chemicals. Salivation, abdominal pain, diarrhea, and convulsions are common symptoms. Atropine given by injection is an antidote which relieves the signs.

Section XX

Useful Information

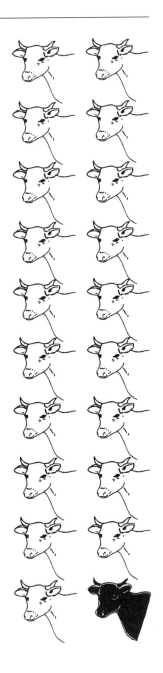

USEFUL INFORMATION

VOLUME: How much space or bulk something has. Used for measuring liquids.

1 teaspoon = 5 cubic centimeters (cc) or 5 milliliters (ml).

3 teaspoons = 1 tablespoon.

1 tablespoon = 15 cc/ml.

2 Tablespoons = 30 cc/ml = One fluid ounce.

8 ounces = 1 cup = 240 cc/ml.

2 cups = 1 pint = 480 cc/ml.

2 pints = 1 quart = 32 fluid ounces.

1 quart = Approx. 1 liter (1000 cc/ml) (1 quart is just a little less than a liter).

4 quarts = 1 gallon = Approx. 4000 cc/ml.

WEIGHTS: How heavy something is.

16 ounces (oz) = one pound (lb).

1 pound = 454 grams (gm).

1000 grams = 1 kilogram (kilo, kg).

1 kilogram = 2.54 pounds.

1 ounce = 28 grams.

1 gram = 1000 mg.

1 grain (gr) = 65 mg.

METRIC MEASUREMENTS

1 milliliter (ml) = 1 cubic centimeter (cc).

1000 ml = 1 liter.

1 gram (gm) = 1000 milligrams (mg).

1 kilogram (kilo, kg) = 2.2 pounds (lb).

INFORMATION ON VITAL SIGNS

Temperature:

Average rectal temperature of the cow is:
38.5 degrees Centigrade or 101.5 degrees Fahrenheit.

Pulse or heart rate:
Average heart rate in the cow is:
60-70 times per minute in the adult animal (higher in the young).

Respiration rate:
Average respiration rate in the cow is:
30 times per minute. (higher in the young).

DEC — 2013

KERSHAW COUNTY LIBRARY

3 3255 00313 889 9